Instant Work-Ups:
A Clinical Guide to Pediatrics

Instant Work-Ups:
A Clinical Guide
to Pediatrics

Theodore X. O'Connell, MD
Program Director, Director of Residency Research Curriculum, Family Medicine
Residency Program, Kaiser Permanente; Partner Physician Southern California
Permanente Medical Group, Woodland Hills, California; Assistant Clinical
Professor, Department of Family Medicine, David Geffen School of
Medicine at UCLA, Los Angeles, California

Jonathan M. Wong, MD
Partner Physician, Southern California Permanente Medical Group,
Woodland Hills, California

Kevin Haggerty, MD
Associate Physician, Southern California Permanente Medical Group,
Woodland Hills, California

Timothy J. Horita, MD
Partner Physician, Southern California Permanente Medical Group, Woodland
Hills, California; Clinical Assistant Professor, Department of Family Medicine,
David Geffen School of Medicine at UCLA, Los Angeles, California

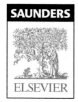

SAUNDERS

ELSEVIER

SAUNDERS
ELSEVIER

1600 John F. Kennedy Blvd.
Ste 1800
Philadelphia, PA 19103-2899

INSTANT WORK-UPS: A Clinical Guide to Pediatrics   ISBN: 978-1-4160-5462-7
Copyright © 2010 by Saunders, an imprint of Elsevier Inc.

Notice

Knowledge and best practice in this field are constantly changing. As new research and experience broaden our knowledge, changes in practice, treatment and drug therapy may become necessary or appropriate. Readers are advised to check the most current information provided (i) on procedures featured or (ii) by the manufacturer of each product to be administered, to verify the recommended dose or formula, the method and duration of administration, and contraindications. It is the responsibility of the practitioner, relying on their own experience and knowledge of the patient, to make diagnoses, to determine dosages and the best treatment for each individual patient, and to take all appropriate safety precautions. To the fullest extent of the law, neither the Publisher nor the Authors assumes any liability for any injury and/or damage to persons or property arising out of or related to any use of the material contained in this book.

The Publisher

Library of Congress Cataloging-in-Publication Data
Instant work-ups : a clinical guide to pediatrics / Theodore X. O'Connell … [et al.]. – 1st ed.
  p. ; cm.
  Includes bibliographical references.
  ISBN 978-1-4160-5462-7
1. Pediatrics–Handbooks, manuals, etc. I. O'Connell, Theodore X. II. Title: Clinical guide to pediatrics.
  [DNLM: 1. Pediatrics–Handbooks. WS 39 I59 2010]
  R–J48.I57 2010
  618.92–dc22   2009011160

Acquisitions Editor: James Merritt
Developmental Editor: Nicole DiCicco
Publishing Services Manager: Joan Sinclair
Project Manager: Sukanthi Sukumar
Design Direction: Louis Forgione
Cover Art:

Working together to grow
libraries in developing countries
www.elsevier.com | www.bookaid.org | www.sabre.org

ELSEVIER   BOOK AID International   Sabre Foundation

Printed in United States
Last digit is the print number: 9 8 7 6 5 4 3 2 1

About the Author

Theodore X. O'Connell, MD, is the Program Director of the Kaiser Permanente Woodland Hills Family Medicine Residency Program where he also directs the residency research curriculum. Dr. O'Connell is a partner in the Southern California Permanente Medical Group and a clinical instructor in the Department of Family Medicine at the David Geffen School of Medicine at UCLA. He is the recipient of numerous clinical, teaching, and research awards. Dr. O'Connell has been published widely as the author of textbook chapters, review books, journal articles, and editorials. He received his medical degree from the University of California, Los Angeles School of Medicine and completed a residency and chief residency at Santa Monica-UCLA Medical Center in Santa Monica, California.

For Nichole
Our children couldn't have a better mother,
And I couldn't ask for a more wonderful wife.
Thank you for being patient and supportive while
allowing me the time to complete this book. I love you.

Preface

The first ideas for this text came from my experiences as a practicing clinician involved in resident and medical student education. Most medical textbooks are oriented on the basis of a known diagnosis. If one wants to learn more about developmental milestones, inborn errors of metabolism, or rheumatic diseases, traditional textbooks can be great sources of information.

However, patients do not come to the clinician labeled with a diagnosis, except for those problems that have been identified previously. Patients instead come with symptoms such as heart murmur, seizure, and chronic diarrhea or with signs such as purpura, neck mass, or scrotal mass. It is the role of the clinician to use the history, physical examination, and selected laboratory or imaging studies to sort out the patient's present symptom or laboratory abnormality and provide a diagnosis.

As I developed my clinical practice, I began creating list of fairly standardized work-ups for common clinical problems. The work-up could then be tailored to each patient based on the patient's medical history and physical examination findings. This process made it simpler for me to initiate work-ups, saved me time in ordering tests, and helped prevent me from forgetting any important components of the work-up.

Over time, I found that many of our residents were carrying my work-ups in their pockets for use with their patients and that colleagues began using them as well. I added background information so that it would be clear why each test was indicated and in which cases additional portions of the work-up might be appropriate. Then one day it occurred to me that there were many more symptoms and clinical problems that could be outlined and explained in a similar format. Furthermore, many other busy clinicians might like to use these quick work-ups to save time in their medical practices.

This text is written for primary care physicians, particularly family physicians and pediatricians, but it will also be useful for residents and medical students. The work-ups outlined in each chapter are suggested courses of action based on the current medical literature. However, they are not a replacement for clinical judgment and should not be uniformly applied to all patients. Every patient is different, and the history and physical examination may indicate a need for more or less evaluation than these work-ups suggest. These work-ups should be viewed as general guidelines to help the busy clinician be exacting and thorough while also being efficient. At the same time, deviating from these work-ups on the basis of clinical judgment is encouraged and expected.

I hope this text eases your practice of medicine while helping you provide the highest quality care to your patients.

Ted O'Connell, MD

Contents

Theodore X. O'Connell

The medical literature uses varied defining criteria for chronic and recurrent abdominal pain. *Chronic abdominal* pain is now usually defined as long-lasting intermittent or constant abdominal pain of at least 3 months' duration. *Recurrent abdominal pain* is defined as at least three bouts of pain, severe enough to affect activities, over a period of at least 3 months. For many years, the term *recurrent abdominal pain* was used to describe all cases without an identified organic cause. It is now agreed that recurrent abdominal pain is a description, not a diagnosis. The exact prevalence of chronic abdominal pain is not clear, but it seems to account for 2% to 4% of all pediatric office visits, and the prevalence increases with age. In boys, the peak incidence occurs between 5 and 6 years of age, whereas girls have two peaks: one between 5 and 6 years of age and another between 9 and 10 years of age.

A complete history and physical examination are the most important components of the evaluation of any child with chronic abdominal pain. The history is used to assess possible organic causes for the abdominal pain as well as psychosocial factors that may be contributing. The HEADSS mnemonic (home life, education level, activities, drug use, sexual activity, suicide ideation/attempts) is a useful tool to screen for psychosocial problems. The history and physical examination can then be augmented by selected laboratory testing, imaging studies, and empiric therapies.

The two broad categories in the differential diagnosis for chronic abdominal pain in children are *organic disorders* and *functional disorders*. In organic disorders, physiologic, structural, or biochemical abnormalities are present. Functional disorders are conditions in which the patient has a variable combination of symptoms without an identifiable structural or biochemical abnormality and for which no specific test exists to establish the diagnosis. Functional gastrointestinal disorders recognized in childhood include functional dyspepsia, irritable bowel syndrome (IBS), functional abdominal pain, abdominal migraine, and aerophagia. The organic and functional categories are not mutually exclusive: both organic and psychological conditions can coexist and interact.

The Rome III diagnostic criteria for **functional dyspepsia** is defined as all of the following symptoms at least once per week for at least 2 months:

1. Persistent or recurrent pain or discomfort centered in the upper abdomen (superior to the umbilicus)
2. Not relieved by defecation or associated with the onset of a change in stool frequency or stool form (i.e., not IBS)
3. No evidence of an inflammatory, anatomic, metabolic, or neoplastic process that explains the subject's symptoms

The Rome III diagnostic criteria for **irritable bowel syndrome** must include all of the following at least once per week for at least 2 months before diagnosis:

1. Abdominal discomfort (an uncomfortable sensation not described as pain) or pain associated with two or more of the following at least 25% of the time:
   a. Improvement with defecation
   b. Onset associated with a change in frequency of stool
   c. Onset associated with a change in form (appearance) of stool
2. No evidence of an inflammatory, anatomic, metabolic, or neoplastic process that explains the subject's symptoms

The Rome III diagnostic criteria for **childhood functional abdominal pain** must include all of the following at least once per week for at least 2 months before diagnosis:

1. Episodic or continuous abdominal pain
2. Insufficient criteria for other functional gastrointestinal disorders
3. No evidence of an inflammatory, anatomic, metabolic, or neoplastic process that explains the subject's symptoms

The diagnosis of childhood functional abdominal pain syndrome must include childhood abdominal pain at least 25% of the time and one or more of the following:

1. Some loss of daily functioning
2. Additional somatic symptoms such as headache, limb pain, or difficulty sleeping

The Rome III diagnostic criteria for **abdominal migraine** require that all of the following symptoms be present two or more times in the preceding 12 months:

1. Paroxysmal episodes of intense, acute periumbilical pain that lasts for 1 hour or longer
2. Intervening periods of usual health lasting weeks to months
3. The pain interferes with normal activities
4. The pain is associated with two or more of the following:
   a. Anorexia
   b. Nausea
   c. Vomiting
   d. Headache
   e. Photophobia
   f. Pallor
5. No evidence of an inflammatory, anatomic, metabolic, or neoplastic process that explains the subject's symptoms

The Rome III diagnostic criteria define **aerophagia** as at least two of the following symptoms occurring at least once per week for at least 2 months:

1. Air swallowing
2. Abdominal distention because of intraluminal air
3. Repetitive belching, increased flatus, or both

Causes of Chronic or Recurrent Abdominal Pain

Abdominal migraine

Abdominal wall pain

Aerophagia

Aminoacidopathies

Anatomic abnormalities

- Intestinal duplication
- Malrotation
- Recurrent intussusception
- Stricture
- Web

Appendicitis

Bowel obstruction

Carbohydrate intolerance (lactose, fructose, sorbitol, sucrase-isomaltase deficiency)

Celiac disease

Crohn's disease

Diabetes

Diverticulitis

Duodenitis

Eosinophilic esophagitis

Eosinophilic gastroenteritis

Esophagitis

Extra abdominal causes

- Myocardial infarction
- Pneumonia or empyema

Familial Mediterranean fever

Functional abdominal pain

Functional dyspepsia

Gastric ulcer

Gastritis

Genitourinary abnormalities
- Hydronephrosis
- Nephrolithiasis
- Ovarian cyst
- Pregnancy or ectopic pregnancy
- Salpingitis
- Ureteropelvic junction obstruction
- Urinary tract infection

Hepatobiliary disease
- Budd-Chiari syndrome
- Cholangitis
- Cholecystitis
- Choledochal cyst
- Hepatitis

Hernia

IBS

Lead toxicity

Malaria

Mesenteric adenitis

Mesenteric ischemia

Pancreatitis

Parasitic infection (*Giardia*)

Peptic ulcer disease

Peritonitis

Splenic abscess

Splenic infarct

Subdiaphragmatic abscess

Ulcerative colitis

Urinary tract infection

Key Historical Features

✓ Onset and course of pain

✓ Location

✓ Intensity

✓ Duration

✓ Frequency

✓ Quality

✓ Radiation

✓ Time of day or night

✓ Nausea or vomiting

✓ Appetite

✓ Diet

✓ Stool pattern and consistency

✓ Blood in stool

✓ Associated symptoms
  - Diaphoresis
  - Dizziness
  - Nausea

✓ Systemic symptoms
  - Weight loss or gain
  - Fever
  - Rashes
  - Joint pain
  - Delayed growth
  - Delayed pubertal development
  - Chronic cough
  - Reactive airway disease
  - Persistent laryngitis
  - Chest pain

✓ Effect of symptoms on activities, school, play, and relationships

✓ Attempted interventions or therapies

✓ Purging behavior

✓ Past medical history

✓ Menstrual history

✓ Past surgical history

✓ Medications

✓ Family history, especially of peptic disease, inflammatory bowel disease, pancreatitis, biliary disease, IBS, or migraine

✓ Social history
  - Travel
  - Stressors
  - Sexual activity and contraception

Key Physical Findings

- ✓ Weight
- ✓ Height
- ✓ Blood pressure
- ✓ Growth velocity
- ✓ Weight-for-height documentation
- ✓ Pubertal stage
- ✓ Complete physical examination
- ✓ Abdominal examination for general appearance, location of tenderness, mass, rebound, distention, psoas sign, liver size, spleen size, kidney size, or ascites. Auscultation for bowel sounds and bruits
- ✓ Back examination for flank tenderness
- ✓ Rectal examination with stool testing for occult blood
- ✓ Pelvic examination if indicated

Suggested Work-Up

Symptom diary	A diary that includes diet, symptoms, and associated features may help to identify potential causes of the patient's symptoms
Complete blood count (CBC) with differential	To evaluate for infection, inflammation, or anemia
Erythrocyte sedimentation	To evaluate for inflammatory processes
Urinalysis and urine culture	To evaluate for urinary tract infection or hematuria
Stool testing for occult blood	To evaluate for gastrointestinal bleeding
Pregnancy test	For girls of reproductive age

Additional Work-Up

Serum electrolytes, creatinine, blood urea nitrogen (BUN), and glucose	To evaluate for a metabolic cause for abdominal pain
Liver enzymes and amylase	To evaluate for liver disease or pancreatitis

Stool culture	If a bacterial infection is suspected
Stool testing for ova and parasites or *Giardia* antigen	If a parasitic or protozoal cause is suspected
Serologic testing for *Helicobacter pylori*	If *H. pylori* infection is suspected
Cultures for sexually transmitted diseases	If risk factors are present in the history or if the physical examination suggests sexually transmitted disease
Carbohydrate breath testing	To evaluate for lactose intolerance
Abdominal and pelvic ultrasonography	Ultrasound typically is one of the first imaging studies used because of its sensitivity for free fluid and the frequency of retroperitoneal disease. Ultrasound is able to inspect the ileum for Crohn's disease as well as adenopathy and chronic features of abscess from fistulas or Meckel's diverticulum
Upper gastrointestinal series with small bowel follow through	If chronic peptic disease or small bowel inflammatory bowel disease is suspected
Abdominal computed tomography (CT) scan	If extraintestinal mass lesions, abscess, or peritoneal disease are suspected, though the radiation exposure must be considered carefully
Upper endoscopy	Rarely indicated as a first-line investigation but useful in diagnosing eosinophilic gastritis, reflux esophagitis, *H. pylori* infection, Crohn's disease, and villous injury in enteropathy
Colonoscopy	May be useful in the evaluation of chronic diarrhea or bleeding
Barium enema	Indicated primarily in the context of obstruction or chronic intussusception

References

1. Subcommittee on Chronic Abdominal Pain. Technical report. Chronic abdominal pain in children. *Pediatrics* 2005;115(3):e370–381.
2. Lake AM. Chronic abdominal pain in childhood: diagnosis and management. *Am Fam Physician* 1999;59:1823–1830.
3. Longstreth GF, Thompson WG, Chey WD, Houghton LA, Mearin F, Spiller RC. Functional bowel disorders. *Gastroenterology* 2006;130:1480.
4. McCollough M, Sharieff GQ. Abdominal pain in children. *Pediatr Clin North Am* 2006;53:107–137.
5. Ramchandani PG, Hotofp M, Sandhu B, Stein A. The epidemiology of recurrent abdominal pain from 2 to 6 years of age: results of a large, population-based study. *Pediatrics* 2005;116:46–50.
6. Rasquin A. Childhood functional gastrointestinal disorders: child/adolescent. *Gastroenterology* 2006;130:1527–1537.
7. Zeiter DK, Hyams JS. Recurrent abdominal pain in children. *Pediatr Clin North Am* 2002;49:53–71.

Timothy J. Horita

Subtle variations in the size and shape of a child's face and head may be difficult to detect, and variations may be the result of normal differences. However, on occasion, these variances can be the result of an underlying pathologic process. It is in these instances that early detection can prompt interventions that can both allay parental anxiety and limit morbidity.

What constitutes a normal head size is based on statistical renderings of morphology. Abnormalities detected more easily by routine screening, measurement, and plotting on graphs that are widely available. Accurate measurement of the occiputofrontal circumference (OFC) is crucial in this regard. Abnormal head or face shapes may vary from the very subtle to the dramatic. Without direct familiarity of the more common syndromes that cause these abnormalities, a health care provider might detect that some abnormality exists without being able to articulate or pinpoint exactly what is outside the norm. Morphologic nomenclature is outlined in Table 2-1.

An understanding of how the skull develops in relation to the bone structure's response to brain structure is vital to this topic. Both genetic and environmental factors strongly influence this interplay. As the neonatal and infant brain greatly expands during normal neurodevelopment, the skull acts as an ever-changing and vital protective structure. Abnormalities of brain development or abnormalities of bony expansion are the primary reasons for abnormal head size and shape.

Term	Meaning	Suture Involved
Dolichocephaly	Long head	Sagittal suture
Scaphocephaly	Keel-shaped head	Sagittal suture
Acrocephaly	Pointed head	Coronal, lambdoid, or all sutures
Brachycephaly	Short head	Coronal suture
Oxycephaly	Tower-shaped head	Coronal, lamboid, or all sutures
Turricephaly	Tower-shaped head	Coronal suture
Trigonocephaly	Triangular-shaped head	Metopic suture
Plagiocephaly	Asymmetric head	Unilateral lambdoid or positional
Kleeblattschadel	Cloverleaf skull	Multiple but not all sutures
Craniofacial dysostosis	Midface deficiency	Craniosynostosis with involvement of cranial base sutures

(From Mooney PM, Siegel MI. *Understanding Craniofacial Anomalies.* New York: Wiley-Liss; 2002:12, with permission.)

Table 2-1. Morphologic Nomenclature in Common Usage

Although the causes of more serious abnormalities require early detection and intervention, even the more benign and common causes can benefit from treatment.

Plagiocephaly (a deformational abnormality of the skull) needs to be recognized as separate from craniosynostosis (premature fusion of growth plates) and abnormalities of brain development. Distinguishing between these entities can be a challenge, but several key features of each are vital to the provider and are outlined in Table 2-2.

Craniosynostosis, the premature fusion of one or more of the cranial sutures (Figure 2-1), can occur as part of a syndrome or as an isolated defect. Craniosynostosis is called "simple" when only one suture is involved and "compound" when two or more sutures are involved. Craniosynostosis is most commonly present at birth but is not always diagnosed when mild. Usually it is diagnosed as a cranial deformity in the first few months of life.

It is important to differentiate lambdoid synostosis from deformational plagiocephaly, which results from local pressure on a specific region of the skull, typically in one occipital region. The number of infants with deformational plagiocephaly has increased, partly as a result of the

	Deformational Plagiocephaly	Craniosynostosis
Frontal bossing	Ipsilateral to posterior flattening	Absent or contralateral to posterior flattening
Posterior bossing	Absent	Contralateral to posterior flattening and parietal in location
Ipsilateral ear	Displaced anteriorly	Displaced posteriorly toward the fused suture
Sutural ridging	Absent	Often present over the suspected suture

Table 2-2. Differences between Plagiocephaly and Craniosynostosis

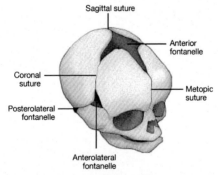

Figure 2-1. Major cranial sutures and fontanelles.
(From Texas Pediatric Surgical Associates, Houston, Texas, with permission.)

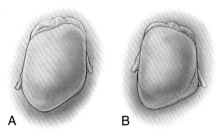

Figure 2-2. Differences between positional plagiocephaly **(A)** and unilamdoid synostosis **(B)**.
(From Gruss JS, Ellenbogen RG, Whelan MF. Lambdoid synostosis and posterior plagiocephaly. In: Lin KY, Ogle RC, Jane JA, eds. *Craniofacial Surgery: Science and Surgical Technique.* Philadelphia: WB Saunders; 2002:242.)

"Back to Sleep" campaign. The diagnosis of deformational plagiocephaly can be made clinically by viewing the infant's head from the top. The differences between deformational plagiocephaly and craniosynostosis are outlined in Figure 2-2. The diagnosis of deformational plagiocephaly is made when the deformations noted in Figure 2-2 are present in an infant who had a typically round head at birth but, a few weeks or months later, the parents notice deformation of head shape.

Medications Associated with Abnormal Head Size and Shape (In Utero Exposure)

- Aminopterin/methotrexate
- Cyclophosphamide
- Ethanol
- Fluconazole
- Methotrexate
- Other environmental teratogens
- Phenytoin
- Radiation exposure
- Retinoids
- Valproate

Causes of Abnormal Head Size and Shape

Microcephaly (OFC <5%)

- Normal variant (by definition 5%) or familial
- Abnormal brain development or delay

- Ischemic encephalopathy
- TORCH (toxoplasmosis, other infections, rubella, cytomegalovirus infection, and herpes simplex virus) exposure
- Craniosynostosis (rare without other skull deformity)

Macrocephaly (OFC >95%)

- Normal variant (by definition 5%) or familial
- Hydrocephalus
- Subdural hematoma
- Brain mass (benign or malignant)
- Syndromic congenital abnormalities
- Nonsyndromic congenital abnormalities

Abnormal Head Shape

- Normal birth molding (newborn)
- Cephalohematoma (newborn)
- Skull or scalp lesion
- Osteomyelitis
- Neoplasm of the brain
- Skull fracture
- Plagiocephaly (nonsynostotic deformation), especially of the occipital skull
- Craniosynostosis
- Syndromic congenital abnormalities
- Nonsyndromic abnormalities
- Rickets
- Hyperthyroidism

Key Historical Features

✓ Abnormal in utero positioning

✓ Oligohydramnios

✓ Multiple gestation

✓ Comprehensive neurodevelopmental history

✓ Milestones reached appropriately

✓ Neurologic symptoms in the older child such as headache, visual disturbance, or unexplained vomiting

✓ Irritability not otherwise explained

✓ Lethargy

✓ Poor feeding or vomiting

✓ Sleeping position

✓ Family history
  • Microcephaly
  • Macrocephaly/hydrocephalus
  • Abnormal head shape or large head size

✓ History of head trauma

✓ Suspicion of abuse or neglect

Key Physical Findings

✓ Accurate measurement of the occipitofrontal circumference

✓ Bulging fontanelle

✓ Funduscopic examination for papilledema

✓ Abnormal positioning of the ears

✓ Asymmetry or other abnormalities of facies

✓ Flattened occiput and ipsilateral bulging frontal skull (suggesting possible plagiocephaly)

✓ Abnormal weight loss or deceleration of growth

✓ Neurologic examination for hypotonia

✓ Other evidence of syndromic dysmorphisms

✓ Palpable suture ridge (with abnormal head size)

✓ Premature or late closure of anterior fontanelle (with abnormal head size)

Suggested Work-Up

Concise plotting of growth curves	For screening purposes and to determine whether microcephaly or macrocephaly is present
Measurement of parents and siblings	To determine whether head size variation is familial
Skull radiographs (anteroposterior and lateral views of the skull) or computed tomography (CT)	To evaluate the sutures in cases of suspected craniosynostosis. The sutures can be identified more accurately on a CT scan, and CT scanning helps in evaluating the brain for structural abnormalities and in excluding other causes of asymmetric vault growth

| Pediatric neurosurgery consultation | Usually indicated in cases of macrocephaly or head deformity |
| Pediatric neurology or genetics consultation | Usually indicated for cases of microcephaly without skull deformity |

Additional Work-Up

Ultrasonography	Can be used to evaluate for ventricular dilatation if the anterior fontanelle is open
Magnetic resonance imaging (MRI)	Preferable if neuroanatomy needs to be visualized well. Can detect cortical and white-matter abnormalities such as degenerative diseases and can document the extent of calvarial masses.
Genetic studies, including karyotyping or genetic screening for syndromic phenotypes	If indicated by history and physical examination. Often deferred until genetics consultation is obtained
Thyroid-stimulating hormone (TSH)	If hyperthyroidism is suspected
Blood urea nitrogen (BUN) and creatinine	If renal failure is suspected (linked to rickets and craniosynostosis)
Vitamin D level	If rickets is suspected (linked to craniosynostosis)

References

1. Delashaw J, Persing J, Jane J. Cranial deformation in craniosynostosis: a new explanation. *Neurosurg Clin North Am* 1991;2:611–620.
2. Dufresne C, Carson B, Zinreich S. *Complex Craniofacial Problems.* New York: Churchill Livingstone; 1992:160.
3. Gruss JS, Ellenbogen RG, Whelan MF. Lambdoid synostosis and posterior plagiocephaly. In: Lin KY, Ogle RC, Jane JA, eds. *Craniofacial Surgery: Science and Surgical Technique.* Philadelphia: WB Saunders; 2002:233–351.
4. Hoyte D. The cranial base in normal and abnormal skull growth. *Neurosurg Clin N Am* 1991;2:515–537.
5. Kiesler J, Ricer R. The abnormal fontanel. *Am Fam Physician* 2003;67:2547–2552.
6. Mooney MP, Siegel MI. *Understanding Craniofacial Anomalies.* New York: Wiley-Liss; 2002:4.
7. Piatt JH Jr. Recognizing neurosurgical conditions in the pediatrician's office. *Pediatr Clin North Am* 2004;51(2):237–270.
8. Ridgway EB, Weiner HL. Skull deformities. *Pediatr Clin North Am* 2004;51(2):359–387.

Theodore X. O'Connell

Every male patient with the acute onset of pain and swelling of the scrotum requires an immediate evaluation to diagnose or exclude testicular torsion. Of the cases of acute painful scrotum, 30% are caused by testicular torsion. Testicular torsion represents a true surgical emergency because the likelihood of testicular salvage decreases as the duration of torsion increases. The rate of testicular salvage is highest with symptoms 6 or fewer hours in duration. In children in whom the duration of symptoms is short and in whom clinical history and physical examination strongly suggest the diagnosis of acute testicular torsion, imaging studies may be bypassed in favor of surgical exploration.

The age of the child may help guide the evaluation. Testicular torsion may occur at any age but is more common during the newborn period and during early puberty. Appendiceal torsion and Henoch-Schönlein purpura are more common in prepubertal boys. Epididymitis is more common in adolescents and young adults.

The abrupt onset of severe pain is characteristic of testicular torsion. Mild to moderate pain that develops over several days is more suggestive of epididymitis or appendiceal torsion. An acute scrotal process may be referred to the abdomen, so any child presenting with an acute abdomen must have a complete genital examination.

Causes of Acute Scrotal Pain

Acute idiopathic scrotal edema

Allergic reaction

Appendiceal torsion

Epididymitis

Henoch-Schönlein purpura

Hydrocele

Inguinal hernia

Insect bite

Orchitis

Testicular torsion

Trauma

- Hematocele (blood within the tunica vaginalis)
- Intratesticular hematoma
- Laceration of the tunica albuginea
- Testicular rupture

Varicocele

Key Historical Features

✓ Onset and duration of pain

✓ Abdominal pain

✓ Nausea or vomiting

✓ Fever

✓ Voiding symptoms such as dysuria, urgency, or frequency

✓ New incontinence

✓ History of trauma

✓ History of acute scrotal pain in the past that resolved after a short time, which may suggest prior testicular torsion with spontaneous detorsion

✓ Past medical history, especially:

  • Congenital genitourinary abnormalities

  • Hydrocele

  • Neurogenic bladder

  • Urethral instrumentation

✓ Past surgical history, especially surgery for undescended testis, hernia, or hydrocele

✓ Sexual activity

Key Physical Findings

✓ Vital signs

✓ Assessment of degree of discomfort

✓ Abdominal examination

✓ Evaluation of the penis and scrotum to determine the degree and laterality of swelling, the presence and location of erythema, the lie of the testicles, and the degree of thickening of the scrotal skin

✓ Evaluation of cremasteric reflex. The presence of an intact cremasteric reflex on the affected side indicates the absence of testicular torsion on that side

✓ Examination of the inguinal canals for hernias, swelling, or erythema

✓ Palpation of the testicles, beginning with the unaffected side

  • Tenderness of the entire testicle is consistent with testicular torsion or orchitis

  • Tenderness limited to the upper pole suggests appendiceal torsion, especially when associated with a hard, tender nodule in this area or a small bluish discoloration over the superior pole of the testicle

- Tenderness over the epididymis (which may be indurated) with a relatively nontender testicle suggests the presence of epididymitis

✓ Skin examination for purpura

Suggested Work-Up

Urinalysis	To evaluate for urinary tract infection. An abnormal urinalysis also may be present in a small number of boys with testicular torsion.
Emergent color Doppler ultrasound	If testicular torsion is considered but is not clear from the history and physical examination
Urgent surgical exploration	If testicular torsion is considered the likely diagnosis on the basis of the history and physical examination

Additional Work-Up

Emergent surgical evaluation	If testicular torsion is found on color Doppler ultrasound on the basis of diminished or absent blood flow to the testicle
Urine culture	If epididymitis is suspected
Urethral culture for gonococcus and *Chlamydia* spp.	If urethral discharge is present
Radioisotope imaging	May be used as an alternative to color Doppler ultrasonography for the evaluation of testicular torsion but does not provide any anatomic data

References

1. Kass EJ, Lundak B. The acute scrotum. *Pediatr Clin North Am* 1997;44:1251–1266.
2. Leslie JA, Cain MP. Pediatric urologic emergencies and urgencies. *Pediatr Clin North Am* 2006;53:513–527.
3. Shalaby-Rana E, Lowe LH, Blask AN, Majd M. Imaging in pediatric urology. *Pediatr Clin North Am* 1997;44:1065–1089.
4. Sheldon CA. The pediatric genitourinary examination. *Pediatr Clin North Am* 2001;48:1339–1380.

Jonathan M. Wong

Anemia is a frequent laboratory abnormality in children, affecting as many as 20% of children in the United States and as many as 80% of children in developing countries. Anemia is defined as a decreased concentration of hemoglobin and red blood cell (RBC) mass compared with age-matched controls. Age-specific blood cell indices are outlined below in Table 4-1.

The physiologic anemia of infancy is often confused with a pathologic condition. During the first weeks of life, erythropoietin synthesis abruptly decreases, resulting in a relative anemia. In the ensuing 6 to 8 weeks, the hemoglobin reaches a low point of 9 to 11 g/dL in term infants. The hemoglobin may reach a low point of 7 to 9 g/dL in premature infants. Erythropoietin production is then stimulated, and the hemoglobin level returns to normal. This physiologic anemia does not require work-up unless it is lower than the expected range.

Anemia varies with sex as well as race. African-American children have a lower normal value than their Caucasian counterparts, and glucose-6-phosphate dehydrogenase (G6PD) deficiency is far more common in male than in female children.

Most children with anemia are asymptomatic and have an abnormal hemoglobin level detected at routine screening. A child may present with pallor, fatigue, or jaundice if the anemia is severe or acute.

Anemia usually results from decreased production of RBCs, increased destruction of RBCs, or blood loss. Erythropoietin is the main hormonal regulator of RBC production. In the fetus, it comes from the monocyte/macrophage system of the liver, and postnatally is produced in the peritubular cells of the kidneys.

Medications Associated with Anemia

Acetylsalicylic acid (in patients with G6PD deficiency)

Antibacterials (in patients with G6PD deficiency)

- Chloramphenicol
- Nalidixic acid
- Nitrofurantoin
- Sulfonamides

Antimalarials (in patients with G6PD deficiency)

- Chloroquine
- Paraquine
- Primaquine
- Quinacrine

Table 4-1. Age-Specific Blood Cell Indices

Age	Hb (g%)[a]	Hct (%)[a]	MCV (fL)[a]	MCHC (g% RBC)[a]	Reticulocytes	WBCs (x10³/mm³)[b]	Platelets (10³/mm³)[b]
26-30 wk gestation[c]	13.4 (11)	41.5 (34.9)	118.2 (106.7)	37.9 (30.6)	–	4.4 (2.7)	254 (180–327)
28 wk	14.5	45	120	31.0	(5–10)	–	275
32 wk	15.0	47	118	32.0	(3–10)	–	290
Term[d] (cord)	16.5 (13.5)	51 (42)	108 (98)	33.0 (30.0)	(3–7)	18.1 (9–30)[e]	290
1–3 day	18.5 (14.5)	56 (45)	108 (95)	33.0 (29.0)	(1.8–4.6)	18.9 (9.4–34)	192
2 wk	16.6 (13.4)	53 (41)	105 (88)	31.4 (28.1)	–	11.4 (5.20)	252
1 mo	13.9 (10.7)	44 (33)	101 (91)	31.8 (28.1)	(0.1–1.7)	10.8 (4–19.5)	–
2 mo	11.2 (9.4)	35 (28)	95 (84)	31.8 (28.3)	–	–	–
6 mo	12.6 (11.1)	36 (31)	76 (68)	35.0 (32.7)	(0.7–2.3)	11.9 (6–17.5)	–
6 mo–2 yr	12.0 (10.5)	36 (33)	78 (70)	33.0 (30.0)	–	10.6 (6–17)	(150–350)
2–6 yr	12.5 (11.5)	37 (34)	81 (75)	34.0 (31.0)	(0.5–1.0)	8.5 (5–15.5)	(150–350)
6–12 yr	13.5 (11.5)	40 (35)	86 (77)	34.0 (31.0)	(0.5–1.0)	8.1 (4.5–13.5)	(150–350)
12–18 yr							
Male	14.5 (13)	43 (36)	88 (78)	34.0 (31.0)	(0.5–1.0)	7.8 (4.5–13.5)	(150–350)
Female	14.0 (12)	41 (37)	80 (78)	34.0 (31.0)	(0.5–1.0)	7.8 (4.5–13.5)	(150–350)
Adult							
Male	15.5 (13.5)	47 (41)	90 (80)	34.0 (31.0)	(0.8–2.5)	7.4 (4.5–11)	(150–350)
Female	14.0 (12)	41 (36)	90 (80)	34.0 (31.0)	(0.8–4.1)	7.4 (4.5–11)	(150–350)

[a]Data are mean (±2 SD); [b]Data are mean (±2 SD); [c]Values are from fetal samplings; [d]<1 mo, capillary hemoglobin exceeds venous: 1 h: 3.6 g difference; 5 day: 2.2 g difference; 3 wk: 1.1 g difference; [e]Mean (95% confidence limits).

Hb, hemoglobin; Hct, hematocrit; MCV, mean corpuscular volume; MCHC, mean corpuscular hemoglobin concentration; WBC, white blood cell count.

Data from Forestier F, et al. Pediatr Res 1896;20:342; Oski FA, Naiman JL. Hematological Problems in the Newborn Infant. Philadelphia: WB Saunders; 1982; Nathan D, Oski FA. Hematology of Infancy and Childhood. Philadelphia: WB Saunders; 1998; Matoth Y, Zaizov R, Varsano I. Acta Paediatr Scand 1971;60:317; and Wintrobe MM. Clinical Hematology. Baltimore: Williams & Williams; 1999.

Aspirin

Chemotherapy agents

Clopidogrel

Human immunodeficiency virus (HIV) medications

Methylene blue (in patients with G6PD deficiency)

Phenacetin (in patients with G6PD deficiency)

Phenazopyridine (in patients with G6PD deficiency)

Probenacid (in patients with G6PD deficiency)

Vitamin K analogues (in patients with G6PD deficiency)

Warfarin

Causes of Anemia

Decreased red cell production

✓ Marrow failure
- Aplastic crisis (e.g., parvovirus B19 infection)
- Diamond-Blackfan syndrome
- Fanconi anemia
- Transient erythroblastopenia of childhood

✓ Impaired erythropoietin production
- Chronic inflammatory diseases
- Hypothyroidism
- Protein malnutrition
- Renal failure

✓ Defects in red cell maturation
- Folate deficiency
- Iron deficiency anemia
- Pure red cell aplasia
- Sideroblastic anemia
- Vitamin B_{12} deficiency

Increased red cell destruction

✓ Extracellular
- Autoimmune hemolytic anemias
- Drugs
- Hemolytic uremic syndrome (HUS)
- Mechanical injury from cardiac valvular defects
- Severe burns
- Toxins

✓ Intracellular
- Enzyme defects (e.g., G6PD deficiency, pyruvate kinase deficiency)
- Hemoglobinopathies (e.g., sickle cell disease)
- Paroxysmal nocturnal hemoglobinuria
- Porphyrias
- Thalassemias

Blood loss
✓ Gastrointestinal (GI) tract
✓ Intra abdominal
✓ Intracranial
✓ Pulmonary

Key Historical Features

✓ Blood loss, including source and amount
✓ Recent infections
✓ Ethnic background
✓ Symptoms
- Fatigue
- Lethargy
- Irritability
- Pica
- Dizziness
- Anorexia
- Abdominal pain
- Early satiety
- Dark urine
- Rectal bleeding
- Bone pain
- Joint swelling
✓ Birth and neonatal history
- Gestational age at birth
- Delivery information
- Neonatal jaundice
- Phototherapy

- Anemia
- Transfusion
- Cephalohematoma
✓ Past medical history
- Chronic medical problems
- Developmental delay
✓ Medications
✓ Allergies
✓ Family history
- Anemia
- Jaundice
- Gallbladder disease or surgery
- Splenectomy
- Autoimmune disease
- Bleeding disorders
✓ Social history
- Dietary history
- Travel
- Toxin and chemical exposure

Key Physical Findings

✓ Vital signs
✓ Measurement of weight, height, and head circumference to evaluate for growth delay
✓ General impression of well-being, noting irritability or pallor
✓ Assessment of developmental stage
✓ Head and neck examination for scleral icterus or glossitis
✓ Cardiopulmonary examination for tachycardia, tachypnea, or murmurs. Acute anemia may present with signs of congestive heart failure or hypovolemia
✓ Abdominal examination for fullness, hepatomegaly, or splenomegaly
✓ Extremity examination for edema or nail bed changes
✓ Skin examination for jaundice
✓ Evaluation for any signs of bleeding

Suggested Work-Up

Complete blood cell count (CBC) evaluation of the mean corpuscular volume (MCV)

When a low hemoglobin level is detected, evaluation of the MCV may be used to classify the anemia further as microcytic, normocytic, or macrocytic. The differential diagnosis of each is presented in Table 4-2

Peripheral smear

Pathologic findings on the smear can indicate the cause of the anemia based on RBC morphology. For example, basophilic stippling is seen in thalassemia and lead poisoning, whereas Howell-Jolly bodies are seen in asplenia, pernicious anemia, and severe iron deficiency anemia

Reticulocyte count

The reticulocyte count helps distinguish a hypoproductive anemia (decreased RBC production) versus a destructive process (increased RBC destruction). A low reticulocyte count may indicate bone marrow disorders or aplastic crisis, whereas a high count generally indicates a hemolytic process or active blood loss

There usually is a natural increase in RBC production in response to anemia. The corrected reticulocyte count is the reticulocyte count × (hematocrit [Hct]/normal Hct). This corrected reticulocyte count is generally >2%. A low count is suggestive of chronic anemia/hemolysis or a marrow problem

Additional Work-Up

If the MCV, peripheral smear, and reticulocyte count do not elucidate the diagnosis, other, more specific lab tests can be performed:

Iron studies (ferritin, iron, total iron-binding capacity [TIBC])

If iron deficiency is suspected, a trial of treatment with iron supplementation followed by a repeat CBC is also reasonable. An increase in hemoglobin levels of greater than 1.0 g/dL by 4 weeks is diagnostic of iron deficiency

Coombs' test	To evaluate for autoimmune hemolytic anemia
G6PD assay	If G6PD deficiency is suspected
Hemoglobin electrophoresis	If a hemoglobinopathy is suspected
LDH, total bilirubin, indirect bilirubin, haptoglobin, and reticulocyte count.	If hemolytic anemia is suspected, LDH and indirect bilirubin levels will increase when there is increased RBC destruction. Haptoglobin is reduced with intravascular and extravascular hemolysis. Reticulocyte count will be high
Direct Coombs' test	If hemolytic anemia is suspected. Tests for the presence of antibody on patient's RBCs
Indirect Coombs test	If hemolytic anemia is suspected. Tests for free autoantibody in the patient's serum after RBC antibody binding sites are saturated
Vitamin B_{12} level	If B_{12} deficiency is suspected
Folic acid level	If folic acid deficiency is suspected
Thyroid stimulating hormone (TSH)	If hypothyroidism is suspected
Osmotic fragility tests	If hereditary spherocytosis is suspected
Bone marrow biopsy	If bone marrow failure or malignancy is suspected or if the diagnosis remains in doubt after thorough evaluation
Red cell enzyme studies	If G6PD deficiency or pyruvate kinase deficiency is suspected
Blood typing and cross-matching	If isoimmune anemia is suspected
Specific viral titers	If Epstein-Barr, cytomegalovirus, or parvovirus B19 infection is suspected

Chest radiograph	If leukemia or congestive heart failure is suspected
Computed tomography (CT) scan	If trauma is suspected in the setting of acute anemia
Esophagogastroduodenscopy and/or colonoscopy	If a GI source of blood loss is suspected
Tagged RBC scan	If cryptogenic bleeding is suspected

Reticulocyte Count	Microcytic Anemia	Nomocytic Anemia	Macrocytic Anemia
Low	Iron deficiency Lead poisioning Chronic disease Aluminum toxicity Copper deficiency Protein malnutrition	Chronic disease RBC aplasia (TEC, infection, drug induced) Malignancy Juvenile rheumatoid arthritis Endocrinopathies Renal failure	Folate deficiency Vitamin B_{12} deficiency Aplastic anemia Congenital bone marrow dysfunction (Diamond-Blackfan or Fanconi syndromes) Drug induced Trisomy 21 Hypothyroidism
Normal	Thalassemia trait Sideroblastic	Acute bleeding Hypersplenism Dyserthropioetic anemia II	-
High	Thalassemia syndromes Hemoglobin C disorders	Antibody-mediated hemolysis Hypersplenism Microangiopathy (HUS, TTP, DIC, Kasabach-Merritt) Membranopathies (spherocytosis, eliptocytosis) Enzyme disorders (G6PD, pyruvate kinase) Hemoglobinopathies	Dyserythropioetic anemia I, III Active hemolysis

DIC, disseminated intravascular coagulation; G6PD, glucose-6-phosphate dehydrogenase; HUS, hemolytic-uremic syndrome; TEC, transient erythroblastopenia of childhood; TTP, thrombotic thrombocytopenic purpura.
Data from Nathan D, Oski FA. *Hematology of Infancy and Childhood.* Philadelphia: WB Saunders; 1988.

Table 4-2. Classification of Anemia

References

1. Irwin JJ, Kirchner JT. Anemia in children. *Am Fam Physician* 2001;64:1379–1386.
2. Robertson J, Shilkofski N. *The Harriet Lane Handbook: A Manual for Pediatric House Officers*, 17th ed. St. Louis: Mosby; 2005:73–104.
3. Segel GB, Hirsh MG, Feig SA. Managing anemia in pediatric office practice: part 1. *Pediatr Rev* 2002;23:75–84.
4. Segel GB, Hirsh MG, Feig SA. Managing anemia in pediatric office practice: part 2. *Pediatr Rev* 2002;23:111–122.

Jonathan M. Wong

An apparent life-threatening event (ALTE) is defined as an episode that is frightening to the observer and is characterized by some combination of apnea, color change, change in muscle tone, choking, or gagging. These episodes may necessitate stimulation or resuscitation to arouse the child and reinitiate regular breathing.

The true incidence of ALTEs is unknown because epidemiologic data are derived from inpatient admissions and emergency rooms, and not all children who have an ALTE are brought in for evaluation. The reported incidence of ALTE is 0.05% to 6%. Most episodes occur in children younger than 1 year, and some studies have implied a peak incidence between 1 week and 2 months of age, with most occurring within the first 10 weeks of life.

The underlying cause of ALTE varies greatly and should be thought of as a manifestation of other conditions. In one half of patients, the cause is discovered either through careful history and physical examination, diagnostic evaluation (see below), or both so that intervention is possible, perhaps preventing future episodes. By default, a specific cause is not found in the remaining cases, placing them in the idiopathic category.

According to one major study of 243 patients, history and physical examination alone yielded a cause 21% of the time, whereas diagnostic tests alone (when history and physical were not elucidative), yielded a cause 14% of the time. This speaks to the importance of a careful history and physical examination while revealing that a shotgun approach to diagnostic testing is not helpful.

The challenge is to manage the immediate event, discern the underlying cause, educate parents and alleviate their concerns, and determine the need for future monitoring. The outcome depends on the subgroup into which the patient falls. For example, patients for whom the ALTE was a heralding event (seizure disorder or neurologic condition) have a higher mortality rate and less than optimal outcome. Mortality data reveal a rate between 0% and 4% between 1972 and 1989.

No clear association has been made between sudden infant death syndrome (SIDS) and ALTEs. The rate of ALTEs has *not* decreased with the "back-to-sleep" program; however, patients who have suffered from an ALTE are at greater risk for sudden death. Follow-up studies have shown no long-term neurodevelopmental, cognitive, or gross motor delays in children who have suffered an ALTE compared with controls.

Hospitalization for observation and work-up is recommended for most children with an ALTE. Criteria have been developed to help determine which children should be hospitalized. These criteria include the need for vigorous stimulation or cardiopulmonary resuscitation (CPR) to arouse the child, any abnormalities in the history or physical examination, or an unreliable home situation.

Medications Associated with ALTE

ALTE can be associated with any prescription, over-the-counter, or herbal medicines. It can be associated with accidental ingestion, intentional ingestion, overdose, or underdosing of therapeutic medications. Some common examples include the following:

- Antiepileptics
- Antipsychotics
- Barbiturates
- Ethylene glycol
- Methanol
- Opioids
- Salicylates
- Salt poisoning

Causes of ALTE

Cardiac Causes (~5%)

- Arrhythmia
- Cardiomyopathy
- Congenital heart disease such as double aortic arch
- Long QT syndrome
- Myocarditis
- Wolff-Parkinson-White syndrome

Child Abuse (<5%)

- Munchausen by proxy (suffocation, intentional salt poisoning, medication overdose, physical abuse, head injury)
- Smothering (intentional or accidental)

Gastrointestinal Causes (most common, up to 50% of diagnosed cases)

- Gastric volvulus
- Gastroesophageal reflux disease (GERD)
- Intussusception
- Swallowing abnormalities

Idiopathic, also known as central apnea (up to 50%)

Infectious Causes

- Sepsis
- Urinary tract infection

Metabolic Abnormalities (<5%)

- Electrolyte disorders
- Endocrine disorders
- Inborn errors of metabolism

Neurologic Causes (~30%)

- Brainstem malformations
- Budd-Chiari malformation
- Central nervous system (CNS) bleeding
- CNS infection (meningitis, encephalitis)
- Febrile seizure
- Hydrocephalus
- Infantile spasm
- Malignancy
- Seizure disorder
- Vasovagal reflex
- Ventriculoperitoneal (VP) shunt malformation

Respiratory Causes (~20%)

- Airway obstruction
- Apnea of prematurity/infancy
- Breath-holding spell
- Bronchiolitis, especially respiratory syncytial virus (RSV)
- Central hypoventilation
- Choking
- Croup
- Foreign body aspiration
- Laryngotracheomalacia
- Mycoplasma
- Obstructive sleep apnea
- Periodic breathing
- Pertussis
- Pneumonia
- Vocal cord abnormalities

Other Causes

- Anaphylaxis
- Carbon monoxide poisoning
- Ethanol ingestion
- Food allergy

Key Historical Features

✓ Evaluation of risk factors for ALTE

- Prematurity (even higher for those with RSV infection or who undergo general anesthesia)
- Rapid feeders
- Frequent coughers
- Choking during feedings
- Male gender
- Previous history of ALTE

✓ Description of the event (best obtained from the most direct witness)

- Duration of event (length of time required to reinstate normal breathing and normal behavior/tone OR length of time of resuscitation)
- Condition of child (awake/asleep)
- Position of child (prone/supine/side)
- Location of child (crib/parent's bed/car seat)
- Surroundings (pillows/bedclothes/blankets)
- Activity at time of event (feeding/coughing/gagging/choking/vomiting)
- Breathing efforts (none/shallow/gasping/increased)
- Color of child and location of any discoloration (pallor/red/purple/blue/peripheral/whole body/circumoral)
- Movement and tone (rigid/tonic-clonic/decreased/floppy)
- Vomiting or sputum production
- Wheeze/stridor/crying
- Interventions (None/gentle stimulation/blowing air in face/vigorous stimulation/mouth-to-mouth/CPR)

✓ Recent symptoms

- Fever
- Poor feeding
- Weight loss

- • Rash
- • Lethargy
- • Sick contacts
✓ Medical history
  - • Prenatal history (use of drugs/alcohol/tobacco during pregnancy)
  - • Prematurity or small for gestational age
  - • Birth history (trauma/hypoxia/presumed sepsis)
  - • Feeding history (gagging/coughing/poor weight gain)
  - • Developmental history
  - • Previous admissions (surgeries, other ALTEs)
  - • Accidents (being dropped/tossed/trauma)
✓ Medications
✓ Allergies
✓ Family history
  - • Congenital problems
  - • Neurologic problems
  - • Neonatal problems
  - • Sudden death
  - • ALTEs
  - • Cardiac arrhythmias
✓ Social history
  - • Home situation
  - • Caregivers
  - • Smoking in home

Key Physical Findings

✓ Vital signs
✓ Height, weight, and head circumference
✓ General impression of the child's well-being
✓ Dysmorphic features or obvious malformations
✓ Neurologic examination, especially muscle tone and reflexes
✓ Appropriateness of developmental stage
✓ Signs of trauma/bruising (retinal hemorrhage, battle sign, raccoon eyes)
✓ Thorough cardiopulmonary examination
✓ Abdominal examination
✓ Genitourinary examination

✓ Musculoskeletal examination

✓ Other areas as directed by the history

Suggested Work-Up

Laboratory and imaging studies should be performed on the basis of history and physical examination. A few baseline tests are generally recommended as a minimum work-up (most likely to lead to a cause for ALTE):

Complete blood cell count (CBC) with differential	To evaluate for infection or anemia
Electrolytes, magnesium, and calcium	To evaluate for electrolyte disturbance or metabolic abnormalities
Serum bicarbonate	To evaluate for hypoxemia or acidosis
Blood urea nitrogen (BUN) and creatinine	To evaluate for dehydration or renal disease
Serum lactate	To evaluate for hypoxemia, toxin exposure (salicylates, ethylene glycol, methanol, ethanol), or hereditary enzyme defects (glycogen storage type I, fatty acid oxidation defects, multiple carboxylase deficiency, methylmalonicaciduria)
Serum glucose	To evaluate for hypoglycemia or hyperglycemia
Urinalysis and urine culture	To evaluate for urinary tract infection
Chest radiographs	To evaluate for infection or cardiomegaly
Electrocardiography (ECG)	To evaluate for arrhythmia or QT abnormalities

Additional Work-Up

The following tests may be indicated based on findings from the history and physical examination:

Blood cultures	If infection/sepsis is suspected
Brain imaging (computed tomography [CT], magnetic resonance imaging [MRI])	To evaluate for trauma, neoplasm, or congenital abnormalities
Nasal swab for RSV	To evaluate for RSV infection
Pertussis culture/serology	To evaluate for pertussis infection
Radioisotope milk scan or esophageal pH	To evaluate for gastroesophageal reflux
Nasopharyngeal aspirate	To evaluate for upper airway infections
Liver function studies	To evaluate for hepatic dysfunction
Lumbar puncture with spinal fluid analysis and cultures	If meningitis is suspected
Stool cultures	If infection is suspected
Urine toxicology screen	If metabolic disorder or accidental/intentional overdose is suspected
Skeletal survey	To evaluate for previous or current fractures
Echocardiogram	To evaluate for valvular dysfunction or structural abnormalities
Pneumogram	To evaluate for breathing problems

References

1. Brand DA, Altman RL, Purtill K, Edwards KS. Yield of diagnostic testing in infants who have had an apparent life-threatening event. *Pediatrics* 2005;115:885–893.
2. Farrell PA, Weiner GM, Lemons JA. SIDS, ALTE, apnea, and the use of home monitors. *Pediatrics in Review* 2002;23:3–9.
3. Hall KL, Zalman B. Evaluation and management of apparent life-threatening events in children. *American Family Physician* 2005;71:2301–2308.

Jonathan M. Wong

Autistic disorder is a pervasive developmental disorder defined behaviorally as a syndrome consisting of abnormal development of social skills (withdrawal, lack of interest in peers), limitations in the use of interactive language (both speech and nonverbal), and sensorimotor deficits (inconsistent responses to environmental stimuli).

The development of impairments is varied and characteristically uneven, resulting in good skills in some areas and poor skills in others. Common impairments include deficiencies in social skills, the use of interactive language, sensorimotor skills, symbolic thinking, protodeclarative pointing, and delays in developmental milestones. These delays in developmental milestones may include slow development, development out of sequence, or regression of previously attained milestones.

Common behaviors in autistic disorder include stereotypic behaviors such as rocking or nonproductive movements of the hands and fingers as well as self-injurious behaviors and self-stimulation. Seizure disorders and mental retardation are also seen frequently in autistic disorder. Table 6-1 below lists the Diagnostic and Statistical Manual (DSM)-IV Diagnostic Criteria for Autistic Disorder.

Autistic disorder occurs at a rate of 5 to 10 in 10,000 persons. The male-to-female ratio is 2:1 in severely handicapped individuals and 4:1 in moderately handicapped individuals. The occurrence rate in siblings is suspected to be from 3% to 7%, representing a 50- to 100-fold increase in risk.

Autism can be thought of as a spectrum of disorders in which patients may range from very highly functioning (e.g., Asperger syndrome) to severely mentally retarded. Most individuals with autism manifest some degree of mental retardation, which typically is moderate in severity.

Medications Associated with Autism

- Thalidomide (intrapartum exposure)
- Valproic acid (intrapartum exposure)

I. A total of six (or more) items from (A), (B), and (C), with at least two from (A), and one each from (B) and (C)
   A. Qualitative impairment in social interaction, as manifested by at least two of the following:
      1. Expression, body posture, and gestures to regulate social interaction
      2. Failure to develop peer relationships appropriate to developmental level
      3. A lack of spontaneous seeking to share enjoyment, interests, or achievements with other people (e.g., by a lack of showing, bringing, or pointing out objects of interest to other people)
      4. Lack of social or emotional reciprocity (*Note:* The description gives the following as examples: not actively participating in simple social play or games, preferring solitary activities, or involving others in activities only as tools or "mechanical" aids
   B. Qualitative impairments in communication as manifested by at least one of the following:
      1. Delay in, or total lack of, the development of spoken language (not accompanied by an attempt to compensate through alternative modes of communication such as gesture or mime)
      2. In individuals with adequate speech, marked impairment in the ability to initiate or sustain a conversation with others
      3. Stereotyped and repetitive use of language or idiosyncratic language
      4. Lack of varied, spontaneous make-believe play or social imitative play appropriate to developmental level
   C. Restricted repetitive and stereotyped patterns of behavior, interests, and activities, as manifested by at least two of the following:
      1. Encompassing preoccupation with one or more stereotyped and restricted patterns of interest that is abnormal either in intensity or focus
      2. Apparently inflexible adherence to specific, nonfunctional routines or rituals
      3. Stereotyped and repetitive motor mannerisms (e.g., hand or finger flapping or twisting or complex whole-body movements)
      4. Persistent preoccupation with parts of objects
II. Delays or abnormal functioning in at least one of the following areas, with onset before age 3 years:
   A. Social interaction
   B. Language used in social communication
   C. Symbolic or imaginative play
III. The disturbance is not better accounted for by Rett's disorder or childhood disintegrative disorder

Table 6-1. DSM-IV Diagnostic Criteria for Autistic Disorder

Causes of Autism

No single cause has been identified for the development of autism. Genetic origins are suspected by twin studies and an increased incidence among siblings. An increased frequency of occurrence is also found in patients with genetic conditions such as fragile X syndrome and tuberous sclerosis. Possible contributing factors include the following:

- Prenatal factors such as fetal alcohol exposure
- Perinatal factors
- Infections
- Inborn errors of metabolism
- Immunology
- Lead poisoning

Key Historical Features

Perinatal History

- Uterine bleeding
- Infections such as rubella
- Delivery history, including prolonged labor or the need for oxygen at birth

Noted Impairments

- Social skills
- Use of interactive language
- Sensorimotor deficiencies
- Symbolic thinking
- Protodeclarative pointing
- Developmental milestones

Typical Behaviors

- Stereotypic behaviors (rocking, nonproductive movements of hands and fingers)
- Self-injurious behaviors
- Self-stimulation

Medical History

- Seizure disorders

Family history, especially of limited cognitive abilities or the presence of dysmorphic features

Medications

Key Physical Findings

Patients with autism typically have a normal appearance, without dysmorphic features. Physical examination would include attention to the following:

- Assessment of gaze
- Protodeclarative pointing (or lack thereof)
- Abnormal motor movements (rocking, stereotypic behaviors)

Suggested Work-Up

Figure 6-1 provides an algorithm for evaluating patients suspected of having autism. The work-up begins with recognition and screening done at well-child visits. Indications for formal developmental evaluation include the following:

- No babbling, pointing, or other gestures by age 12 months
- No single words by age 16 months
- No two-word spontaneous phrases by age 24 months
- Loss of previously learned language or social skills at any age
- Any parental concern about delayed speech and language development, typically noticed at about age 18 months

A number of resources are available for screening, such as the following:

- Checklist for Autism in Toddlers (CHAT)
- Child Developmental Inventory (CDI)
- Denver II Developmental Screening Test
- Parents' Evaluation of Developmental Status (PEDS)
- Pervasive Developmental Disorders Screening Test (PDDST)

Additional Work-Up

Referral to an appropriate developmental disorders center is appropriate if the diagnosis of autism spectrum disorder is entertained. A medical evaluation should also be performed in certain situations to exclude other etiologies of symptoms:

Genetic testing	If indicated by family history
Wood's lamp examination of skin to identify depigmented macules	If tuberous sclerosis is suspected
Lead level	If lead poisoning is suspected
Metabolic screening	If an inborn error of metabolism is suspected
Electroencephalography	If seizure disorder is suspected
Central nervous system (CNS) imaging	If malignancy, hemorrhage, infection, or inflammation is suspected
Formal hearing evaluation	If there is any suspicion of hearing deficit because deafness and profound hearing loss can mimic autism
Vision screening	If any visual disturbance is suspected

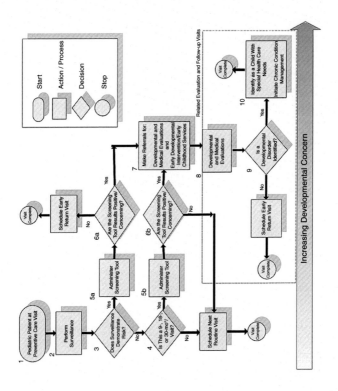

Figure 6-1. Developmental surveillance and screening algorithm within a pediatric preventive care visit. Because the 30-month visit is not yet a part of the preventive care system and is often not reimbursable by third-party payers at this time, developmental screening can be performed at age 24 months.

1. Pediatric Patient at Preventive Care Visit. Developmental concerns should be included as one of several health topics addressed at each pediatric preventive care visit throughout the first 5 years of life.

2. Perform Surveillance. *Developmental surveillance* is a flexible, longitudinal, continuous, and cumulative process whereby knowledgeable health care professionals identify children who may have developmental problems. Developmental surveillance has five components: (a) eliciting and attending to the parents' concerns about their child's development, (b) documenting and maintaining a developmental history, (c) making accurate observations of the child, (d) identifying the risk and protective factors, and (e) maintaining an accurate record and documenting the process and findings.

3. Does Surveillance Demonstrate Risk? The concerns of both parents and child health professionals should be included in determining whether surveillance suggests the child may be at risk of developmental delay. If either parents or the child health professional express concern about the child's development, a developmental screening to specifically address the concern should be conducted.

4. Is This a 9-, 18-, or 30-Month Visit? All children should receive developmental screening using a standardized test. In the absence of established risk factors or parental or provider concerns, a general developmental screen is recommended at the 9-, 18-, and 30-month visits. Additionally, autism-specific screening is recommended for all children at the 18-month visit.

5a and 5b. Administer Screening Tool. *Developmental screening* is the administration of a brief standardized tool that aids in the identification of children at risk of a developmental disorder. Developmental screening that targets the area of concern is indicated whenever a problem is identified during developmental surveillance.

6a and 6b. Are the Screening Tool Results Positive or Cause of Concern? When the results of the periodic screening tool are normal, the child health professional can inform the parents and continue with other aspects of the preventive visit. When a screening tool is administered as a result of concerns about development, an early return visit to provide additional developmental surveillance should be scheduled even if the screening tool results do not indicate a risk of delay.

(Continued)

Figure 6-1. Continued

7-8. Make Referrals for Developmental and Medical Evaluations and Early Developmental Intervention/Early Childhood Services (7). Developmental and Medical Evaluations. (8). If screening results warrant concern, the child should be scheduled for developmental and medical evaluations. *Developmental evaluation* is aimed at identifying the specific developmental disorder or disorders affecting the child. In addition to the developmental evaluation, a *medical diagnostic evaluation* to identify any underlying causes should be undertaken. *Early developmental intervention/early childhood services* can be particularly valuable when a child is first identified to be at high risk of delayed development because these programs often provide evaluation services and can offer other services to the child and family even before an evaluation is complete. Establishing an effective and efficient partnership with early childhood professionals is an important component of successful care coordination for children.

9. Is a Developmental Disorder Identified? If a developmental disorder is identified, the child should be identified as a child with special health care needs, and chronic condition management should be initiated (see no. 10 to follow). If a developmental disorder is not identified through medical and developmental evaluation, the child should be scheduled for an early return visit for further surveillance. More frequent visits, with particular attention paid to areas of concern, will allow the child to be promptly referred for further evaluation if any further evidence of delayed development or a specific disorder emerges.

10. Identification of a Child With Special Health Care Needs. Initial Chronic Condition Management. When a child is discovered to have a significant developmental disorder, that child becomes one with special health care needs, even if that child does not have a specific disease etiology identified. Such a child should be identified by the medical home for appropriate chronic condition management and regular monitoring and entered into the practice's registry of children and youth with special health care needs. (From Council on Children with Disabilities, Section on Developmental Behavioral Pediatrics, Bright Futures Steering Committee and Medical Home Initiatives for Children with Special Needs Project Advisory Committee. Identifying infants and young children with developmental disorders in the medical home: an algorithm for developmental surveillance and screening. *Pediatrics* 2006;118:405–420, with permission.)

References
1. American Psychiatric Association. *Diagnostic and Statistical Manual of Mental Disorders DSM-IV*, 4th ed. Washington, DC: American Psychiatric Association; 1994.
2. Council on Children with Disabilities, Section on Developmental Behavioral Pediatrics, Bright Futures Steering Committee and Medical Home Initiatives for Children with Special Needs Project Advisory Committee. Identifying infants and young children with developmental disorders in the medical home: an algorithm for developmental surveillance and screening. *Pediatrics* 2006;118:405–420.
3. Juul-Dam N, Townsend J, Courchesne E. Prenatal, perinatal, and neonatal factors in autism, pervasive developmental disorder-not otherwise specified, and the general population. *Pediatrics* 2001;107:1–6.
4. Prater CD, Zylstra RG. Autism: a medical primer. *Am Fam Physician* 2002;66:1667–1674.

Theodore X. O'Connell

When a child presents with bruising or bleeding, the challenge for the physician is to ascertain whether the patient's symptoms are appropriate to the hemostatic stress or whether further investigation of an underlying disorder is warranted. The main differential diagnoses are physiologic or accidental bleeding, nonaccidental injury, or a bleeding diathesis. The target of further investigation should be patients with bruising over the trunk, neck, or face, regardless of limb or mucosal bleeding, those with excessive blood loss after minor surgery, or a positive family history.

Bruising caused by accidental injury is common around the age of 1 year, when most infants have started cruising. As a guideline, normal bruising is restricted to the lower limbs; is not associated with petechiae, purpura, or mucosal bleeding; and the family history is negative. Child abuse should be suspected if there is significant bruising or bleeding with no history of trauma or a history inconsistent with the severity of injury. However, in a child with a bleeding diathesis, the child may have bruising or bleeding without a history of trauma. If a child has bruising in a recognizable pattern such as a belt or hand, then suspected abuse must be reported regardless of the outcome of laboratory tests.

Abnormal bleeding or bruising may cause significant anxiety for the patient and may be a sign of a serious inherited or acquired disorder. A history of bleeding following dental extraction, minor surgery, or childbirth suggests an underlying hemostatic disorder. Bleeding that is severe enough to require a blood transfusion merits particular attention. A family history of bleeding abnormalities suggests an inherited systemic disorder, such as von Willebrand disease.

Bleeding from a platelet disorder typically is localized to superficial sites such as the skin or mucous membranes and usually is easily controlled. However, bleeding from hemostatic or plasma coagulation defects may occur hours or days after injury and is difficult to control with local measures. This type of bleeding often occurs into muscles, joints, or body cavities.

Immune thrombocytopenic purpura is the most common hemostatic disorder of childhood to present with easy bruising and is usually associated with petechiae, purpura, and mucosal bleeding. Autosomal dominantly inherited von Willebrand disease is the most common congenital disorder of hemostasis. It often presents with easy bruising as the sole symptom, though mucosal bleeding is common. Purpura and petechiae are not common. Mild hemophilia A (factor VIII deficiency) and B (factor IX deficiency) are much less common but may present with symptoms similar to those of von Willebrand disease. Moderate and severe hemophilia A or B present in infancy with atypical bruising and later with hemarthrosis. Family history is absent in the 30% of sporadic hemophilia.

Initial laboratory tests are outlined below. It is important that results are compared against age-specific ranges because test results and coagulation factor levels vary with age. The pattern of abnormalities obtained using first line tests in association with the clinical presentation and history may indicate an underlying disorder (Table 7-1). However, some significant bleeding disorders may have normal test results. Conversely, some abnormal results are not associated with bleeding.

A thorough history is the most important step in establishing the presence of a hemostatic disorder and in guiding initial laboratory testing. Figure 7-1 provides an approach to investigation of easy bruising or bleeding.

Test Results	Differential Diagnosis	Possible Follow-up Laboratory Studies
PT normal aPTT normal Platelet count normal	Von Willebrand disease Platelet function disorder Factor XIII deficiency Fibrinolytic defect	PFA-100 Von Willebrand studies Urea clot lysis test Euglobulin clot lysis Alpha-2-antiplasmin, PAI-1, TPA
PT normal aPTT prolonged Platelet count normal	PTT inhibitor Von Willebrand disease Hemophilia A or B Factor XI deficiency Heparin contamination	PTT mixing study Factor assays (VIII, IX, XI) Von Willebrand studies Thrombin time/reptilase time
PT prolonged aPTT normal Platelet count normal	PT inhibitor Vitamin K deficiency Warfarin Factor VII deficiency	PT mixing study Factor assays (II, VII, IX, X)
PT prolonged aPTT prolonged Platelet count normal	Circulating inhibitor Liver dysfunction Vitamin K deficiency Factor deficiency (II, V, X, or fibrinogen) Dysfibrinogenemia	PT/PTT mixing studies Thrombin time/reptilase time Fibrinogen Factor assays
PT prolonged aPTT prolonged Platelet count low	DIC Liver dysfunction Kasabach-Merritt syndrome	Thrombin time Fibrinogen Factor assays D-dimers
PT normal aPTT normal Platelet count low	Acute ITP Chronic ITP Collagen vascular disease Early bone marrow Failure syndrome	— Antinuclear antibodies Anticardiolpin antibodies Direct antiglobulin test Serum immunoglobulin levels Serum complement levels Tests for *Helicobacter pylori* Von Willebrand factor multiermeric analysis Bone marrow aspirate Marrow chromosomal analysis

aPTT, activated partial thromboplastin time; DIC, disseminated intravascular coagulation; ITP, immune thrombocytopenia purpura; PAI-1, plasminogen activator inhibitor-1; PT, prothrombin time; TCT, thrombin clot time; TPA, tissue plasminogen activator. From Allen GA, Glader B. Approach to the bleeding child. *Pediatr Clin North Am* 2002;49:1239–1256, with permission.

Table 7-1. Patterns of Coagulation Results and the Differential Diagnosis

Medications Associated with Bleeding

- Abcixcimab
- Aspirin
- Chemotherapeutic agents
- Clopidogrel
- Dalteparin
- Enoxaparin
- Eptifibatide
- Heparin
- Nonsteroidal anti inflammatory drugs
- Phenytoin
- Quinine
- Recombinant t-PAs (Activase and Retavase)
- Steroid inhalers
- Ticlopidine
- Tinzaparin
- Tirofiban
- Urokinase
- Warfarin

Causes of Bleeding

- Acquired factor VIII inhibitors
- Acute leukemia
- Adenocarcinoma
- Afibrinogenemia
- α_2-antiplasmin deficiency
- Amegakaryocyctic thrombocytopenia
- Aplastic anemia
- Bernard-Soulier disease
- Bone marrow failure
- Celiac disease
- Chronic renal failure
- Congenital factor deficiencies
- Disseminated intravascular coagulation
- Drug related thrombocytopenia
- Dysfibrinogenemia
- Ehlers-Danlos syndrome

- Fanconi's anemia
- Fat embolism
- Glanzmann's disease
- HELLP (hemolysis, elevated liver enzymes, and low platelet count) syndrome
- Hemolytic uremic syndrome
- Hemophilia A
- Hemophilia B
- Hemorrhagic disease of the newborn
- Henoch-Schönlein purpura
- Heparin-induced thrombocytopenia
- Human immunodeficiency virus (HIV) infection
- Hypofibrinogenemia
- Idiopathic thrombocytopenic purpura (ITP)
- Leukemia
- Liver disease
- Lyme disease
- Lymphoma
- Malabsorption
- Marfan's syndrome
- May-Hegglin syndrome
- Medications
- Plasminogen activator inhibitor-1 deficiency
- Platelet storage pool disorder
- Post-transfusion purpura syndrome
- Rat poison ingestion (superwarfarins)
- Scott's syndrome
- Sepsis, especially meningococcal
- Storage pool disease
- Systemic lupus erythematosus
- Thrombocytopenia
- Thrombotic thrombocytopenic purpura
- Viral infections
- Vitamin C deficiency
- Vitamin K deficiency
- von Willebrand disease
- Wiskott-Aldrich syndrome

Key Historical Features

✓ How the injury occurred

✓ Duration of the symptoms

✓ Mucous membrane bleeding (menorrhagia, epistaxis, gum bleeding)

✓ Bleeding response to injury such as a bitten tongue

✓ Bleeding into soft tissues such as muscles and joints

✓ Excessive bleeding during surgical procedures (circumcision, tonsillectomy, tooth extraction), fractures, or serious injuries

✓ History of cephalohematoma, unexpected bleeding from the umbilical stump, or bruising after intramuscular injections

✓ Past medical history

✓ Past surgical history

✓ Menstrual and obstetric history in female patients

✓ Medications

✓ Family history of bleeding, including grandparents and the extended family

✓ Details of ethnic origin and consanguinity

Key Physical Findings

✓ General examination for evidence of systemic disease

✓ Epistaxis or bleeding from the gums

✓ Evaluation of the skin for purpura, ecchymoses, or hematomas

✓ Distribution and size of the bruises

✓ Accompanying tissue swelling or abrasion

✓ Lymphadenopathy

✓ Hepatomegaly

✓ Splenomegaly

✓ Evidence of bleeding into muscles or joints

Suggested Work-Up

Complete blood cell count (CBC)	To evaluate for thrombocytopenia and anemia
Peripheral blood smear	To evaluate the cell lines and confirm thrombocytopenia

Prothrombin time (PT)	To evaluate plasma coagulation function
Activated partial thromboplastin time (aPTT)	To evaluate plasma coagulation function
Fibrinogen measurement	To evaluate the functional activity of fibrinogen

Additional Work-Up

Factor VIII, factor IX, von Willebrand factor antigen and activity (Ristocetin cofactor)	Recommended in all cases of non-accidental injury
Mixing study	To evaluate an abnormal PT or aPTT. Normalization of the PT or aPTT following a mixing study indicates a factor deficiency
Coagulation-factor assays (factors VIII, IX, and XI)	Indicated when a factor deficiency is suggested by mixing studies or family history
Factor VII assay	If there is an isolated prolongation of the PT to evaluate for vitamin K deficiency or liver disease
Thrombin time and reptilase time	Indicated if there is an isolated prolongation of the aPTT and heparin contamination from the catheter is suspected. Prolongation of the thrombin time with normal reptilase time is suggestive of heparin contamination. If both the thrombin time and reptilase time are prolonged, the most likely cause is a low fibrinogen concentration
Thrombin time	Used when both the PT and aPTT are prolonged to test for fibrinogen conversion to fibrin. When the thrombin time is prolonged, it signifies low fibrinogen activity, the presence of fibrin split products, or heparin contamination

Factor VIII, von Willebrand factor antigen, von Willebrand factor activity (ristocetin cofactor assay), and factor IX assay	If von Willebrand disease is suspected
PFA-100 platelet function screen	A newer substitute for the bleeding time. The time to occlusion is prolonged in patients with most types of von Willebrand disease and some platelet disorders
PT, aPTT, thromboplastin time, thrombin time, platelet count, factor VIII assay, factor V assay, fibrinogen, and D-dimer	If disseminated intravascular coagulation is suspected

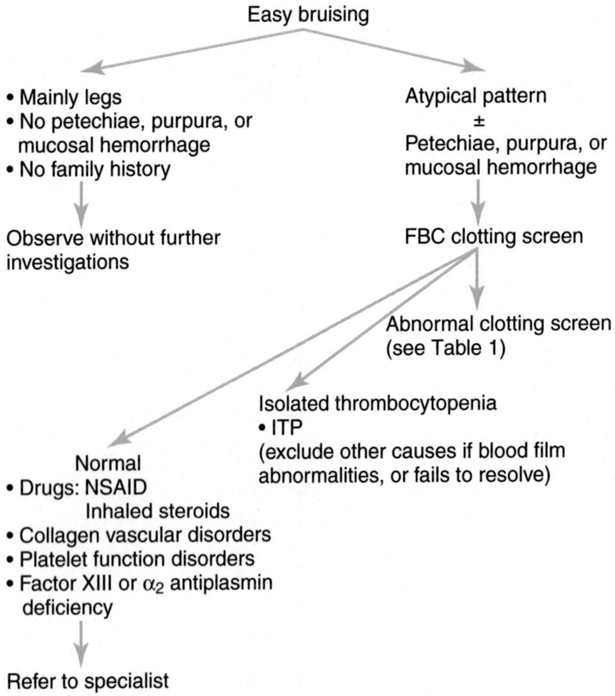

Easy bruising

- Mainly legs
- No petechiae, purpura, or mucosal hemorrhage
- No family history

Observe without further investigations

Atypical pattern
±
Petechiae, purpura, or mucosal hemorrhage

FBC clotting screen

Abnormal clotting screen
(see Table 1)

Isolated thrombocytopenia
- ITP
(exclude other causes if blood film abnormalities, or fails to resolve)

Normal
- Drugs: NSAID
  Inhaled steroids
- Collagen vascular disorders
- Platelet function disorders
- Factor XIII or α_2 antiplasmin deficiency

Refer to specialist

Figure 7-1. An approach to investigation of easy bruising or bleeding. (From Vora A, Makris M. An approach to investigation of easy bruising. *Arch Dis Child* 2001;84:488–491, with permission.)

References

1. Allen GA, Glader B. Approach to the bleeding child. *Pediatr Clin North Am* 2002;49: 1239–1256.
2. Ewenstein BM. The pathophysiology of bleeding disorders presenting as abnormal uterine bleeding. *Am J Obstet Gynecol* 1996;175:770–777.
3. Handin RI. Bleeding and thrombosis. In: Isselbacher KJ, Braunwald E, Wilson JD, eds. *Harrison's Textbook of Internal Medicine.* 13th ed. New York: McGraw-Hill; 1994:317–322.
4. Lusher JM. Screening and diagnosis of coagulation disorders. *Am J Obstet Gynecol* 1996;175:778–783.
5. McKenna R. Abnormal coagulation in the postoperative period contributing to excessive bleeding. *Med Clin North Am* 2001;85:1277–1310.
6. Thomas AE. The bleeding child; is it NAI? *Arch Dis Child* 2004;89:1163–1167.
7. Vora A, Makris M. An approach to investigation of easy bruising. *Arch Dis Child* 2001;84: 488–491.

Theodore X. O'Connell

Lumbar puncture (LP) is a commonly performed procedure in pediatrics, used most commonly to evaluate for the presence of meningitis. Commonly performed tests on cerebrospinal fluid (CSF) include protein and glucose levels, cell counts and differential, microscopic examination, and culture. Additional tests—such as opening pressure, supernatant color, latex agglutination, and polymerase chain reaction—also may be performed.

Protein concentrations usually are elevated in patients with bacterial meningitis. Values less than 40 mg/dL are considered normal in infants and children. The CSF protein may be elevated in many processes, including infectious, immunologic, vascular, and degenerative diseases as well as tumors of the brain and spinal cord. The CSF protein may be increased after a bloody tap by approximately 1 mg/dL for every 1000 mm^3. Values greater than 100 mg/dL suggest that bacterial infection is present. However, protein concentrations of more than 100 to 120 mg/dL commonly are observed in healthy, uninfected newborn infants, especially premature infants.

In most patients with bacterial meningitis, the CSF **glucose** concentration is low as a result of increased metabolic demands. A CSF glucose concentration that is less than half the simultaneously obtained blood glucose concentration usually is considered abnormal.

Normal **white blood cell (WBC) count** values depend on the patient's age. In patients with acute bacterial meningitis, the cell count can be extremely variable, but it is usually in the range of 1000 to 5000 leukocytes/mm^3. However, very early in the illness, the cell count may be normal despite a positive CSF culture. Polymorphonuclear (PMN) cells are always abnormal in a child, but 1 to 2/mm^3 may be present in a normal neonate. An elevated PMN count suggests bacterial meningitis or the early phase of an aseptic meningitis. CSF lymphocytes indicates aseptic, tuberculous, or fungal meningitis; demyelinating diseases; brain or spinal cord tumor; immunologic disorders (including collagen vascular diseases); and chemical irritation (post myelogram, intrathecal methotrexate).

Normal CSF contains no **red blood cells** (RBCs). The presence of RBCs indicates a traumatic tap or a subarachnoid hemorrhage. Progressive clearing of blood CSF is noted during collection of the fluid in the case of a traumatic lumbar puncture.

The probability of seeing bacteria on a Gram-stained CSF preparation is dependent on the number of organisms present. The sensitivity is approximately 80% in a properly prepared smear but is lower when *Listeria monocytogenes* is the cause of meningitis.

Culture should be performed routinely on all spinal fluid specimens, even those that are grossly normal or have normal leukocyte count. The yield of CSF culture is lower in patients previously treated with antibiotics.

The mean opening lumbar **CSF pressure** is variable, depending on the age of the child. These pressures are outlined in Table 8-1. Opening pressures may exceed 150 to 200 mm H_2O when bacterial meningitis is present.

Latex agglutination allows rapid detection of bacterial antigens in CSF. Because false positives lead to unnecessary treatment, latex agglutination is not routinely used today. A positive antigen test result is usually meaningful, but a negative test result is unreliable for excluding a diagnosis of bacterial meningitis. Latex agglutination can be useful in partially treated meningitis

	WBC Count	**Mean % PMNs**
Preterm	0–25 WBCs/mm³	57%
Term	0–22 WBCs/mm³	61%
Child	0–7 WBCs/mm³	5%
Glucose		
Preterm	24–63 mg/dL	1.3–3.5 mmol/L
Term	34–119 mg/dL	1.9–6.6 mmol/L
Child	40–80 mg/dL	2.2–4.4 mmol/L
CSF Glucose/Blood Glucose		
Preterm	55%–105%	
Term	44%–128%	
Child	50%	
Lactic Acid Dehydrogenase		
Normal range	5–30 U/L (or about 10% of serum value)	
Myelin Basic Protein	<4 ng/mL	
Opening Pressure		
(Lateral recumbent)		
Newborn	8–11 cmH₂O	
Infant/Child	<20 cmH₂O	
Respiratory Variations	0.5–1 cmH₂O	
Protein		
Preterm	65–150 mg/dL	0.65–1.5 g/L
Term	20–170 mg/dL	0.20–1.7 g/L
Child	5–40 mg/dL	0.05–0.40 g/L

CSF, cerebrospinal fluid; PMNs, polymorphonuclear lymphocytes; WBC, white blood cell. Modified from Oski FA: *Principles and Practice of Pediatrics*, 3rd ed. Philadelphia: JB Lippincott, 1999:1284–1295.

Table 8-1. Evaluation of Cerebrospinal Fluid

cases where cultures might not yield an organism. Latex agglutination also may be helpful in cases of suspected bacterial meningitis if the initial Gram stain and bacterial culture are negative after 48 hours.

Polymerase chain reaction (PCR) has been especially useful in the diagnosis of viral meningitis. PCR can be used to diagnose infection with enteroviruses, herpes simplex virus, varicella zoster virus, human herpes virus-6, Epstein-Barr virus, cytomegalovirus, arboviruses (California encephalitis group, Japanese encephalitis, West Nile virus, dengue fever virus types 1 to 4, and yellow fever virus).

Contraindications for performing an LP include (1) elevated intracranial pressure due to a suspected mass lesion of the brain or spinal cord, (2) symptoms and signs of pending cerebral herniation in a child with probable meningitis, (3) critical illness (on rare occasions), (4) skin infection at the site of the LP, and (5) thrombocytopenia.

Examination of the cerebrospinal fluid of a patient with acute bacterial meningitis characteristically reveals the following: (1) a cloudy appearance, (2) an increased WBC count with a polymorphonuclear predominance, (3) a low glucose concentration in relation to the serum glucose concentration, (4) an elevated protein concentration, (5) a smear and culture positive for the causative microorganism, and (6) a high manometric pressure. Table 8-2 shows the CSF findings in patients with bacterial meningitis.

The spinal fluid in children with aseptic or proven viral meningitis characteristically shows an increase in lymphocytes and a normal or slightly decreased glucose concentration with a slightly elevated protein concentration. If the CSF is obtained early in the disease process, a large number of PMN cells may be present. A repeat lumbar puncture 24 to 48 hours later can demonstrate the typical lymphocyte predominance.

Finding	Neonates[†]		Infants and Children	
	Normal	Abnormal	Normal	Abnormal
Leukocyte count (cells/μL)	<30	>100	<10w	>1000
Polymorphonuclear (%)	<60	>80	<10	>60-80
Protein (mg/dL)	<170	>200	<40	>100
CSF/blood glucose ratio	>0.6	<0.5	>0.5	<0.4
Manometric pressure (mm H$_2$O)	<60	>100	<90	>150

*Patients with aseptic meningitis can have CSF findings that are indeterminate or fit in the abnormal category.
†Normal values may be different in very-low-birth weight infants.

Table 8-2. Normal and Characteristic Abnormal Cerebrospinal (CSF) Findings in Pediatric Age Groups with or without Bacterial Meningitis*

PCR can provide a specific diagnosis within hours, especially for herpes virus and enteroviruses.

Tuberculous meningitis can be clinically indistinguishable from acute bacterial meningitis. The diagnosis of tuberculous meningitis can be established by (1) an increase in the number of CSF leukocytes, usually from 50 to 500 cells/mm^3, with a lymphocyte predominance, low glucose concentration, very elevated protein concentration, and a culture negative for the usual pathogenic organisms but subsequently positive for tubercle bacilli; (2) a positive tuberculin skin test; (3) chest radiographs showing evidence of a tuberculous lesion; and (4) a positive history of contact with an active case of tuberculosis.

Most infectious causes of chronic meningitis elicit similar CSF abnormalities: a mildly elevated protein concentration, a normal glucose level, and fewer than 500 WBCs/mm^3 with lymphocyte predominance. Table 8-3 outlines distinctive patterns of leukocyte predominance that may aid diagnosis.

Causative Agent	Predominant Leukocytes in CSF		
	Lymphocytes	**Neutrophils**	**Eosinophils**
Bacteria	Mycobacterium tuberculosis Treponema pallidum Borrelia spp. Brucella spp.	Nocardia spp. Actinomyces spp. Brucella spp. Leptospira spp.	M. tuberculosis T. pallidum
Fungi	All	All	Coccidioides spp.
Parasite	Taenia spp. Toxoplasma spp.	Entamoeba histolytica	Angiostrongylus spp. Taenia solium Baylisascaris spp.
Viruses	Lymphocytic choriomeningitis CMV	CMV*	
Other	Parameningeal focus* Sarcoidosis* Chronic idiopathic meningitis Malignant process Behçet disease	Suppurative parameningeal focus* Systemic lupus erythematosus Chemical meningitis Drug hypersensitivity	Hodgkin disease Chemical meningitis Drug hypersensitivity

AIDS, acquired immunodeficiency syndrome; CMV, cytomegalovirus.
*In AIDS patients.
From Yogev R. Chronic meningitis. In: Long SS, Pickering LK, Prober CG, eds. *Principles and Practice of Pediatric Infectious Diseases,* 2nd ed. Philadelphia: Churchill Livingstone; 2003:274–306.

Table 8-3. Predominant Leukocyte Found in Cerebrospinal Fluid (CSF) for Various Causes of Chronic Meningitis

Suggested Work-Up

CSF evaluation:	See preceding text
Protein	
Glucose	
Cell counts and differential	
Gram stain	
Culture	
Blood culture	Should be performed if meningitis is suspected, especially if antibiotics will be started empirically before examination of CSF

Additional Work-Up

CSF opening pressure	See preceding text
CSF latex agglutination	See preceding text
CSF PCR:	As clinically indicated (see preceding text)
Enteroviruses	
Herpes simplex virus (HSV)	
Varicella-zoster virus (VZV)	
Human herpes virus-6 (HHV-6)	
Epstein-Barr virus (HBV)	
Cytomegalovirus (CMV)	
California encephalitis group	
Japanese encephalitis (JE)	
West Nile virus	
Dengue fever virus types 1-4	
Yellow fever virus	
CSF oligoclonal bands	If multiple sclerosis is suspected
CSF lactate, amino acids, and endolase	If metabolic diseases are suspected

References

1. Prober CG. Central nervous system infections. In: Behrman RE, Kliegman RM, Jenson HB, eds. *Nelson Textbook of Pediatrics*, 17th ed. Philadelphia: WB Saunders; 2004: 1980–1981.

2. Robertson J, Shilkofski N, eds. *Johns Hopkins: The Harriet Lane Handbook: A Manual for Pediatric House Officers*, 17th ed. Philadelphia: Mosby; 2005.

3. Sáez-Llorens X, McCracken GH. Meningitis. In: Gershon AA, Hotez PJ, Katz SL, eds. *Krugman's Infectious Diseases of Children*, 11th ed. Philadelphia: Mosby; 2004:377–379, 864–8.

4. Seehusen DA, Reeves MM, Fomin DA. Cerebrospinal fluid analysis. *Am Fam Physician* 2003;68:1103–1108.

5. Yogev R. Chronic meningitis. In: Long SS, Pickering LK, Prober CG, eds. *Principles and Practice of Pediatric Infectious Disease*, 2nd ed. Philadelphia: Churchill Livingstone; 2003: 274–306.

Theodore X. O'Connell

Chest pain in children provokes considerable anxiety for patients and parents. Fortunately, several prospective studies have demonstrated that chest pain in the pediatric age group overwhelmingly is benign. Several organ systems have the potential to cause pain localizing to the thorax. The most common is the musculoskeletal system, where pain can originate from muscle bodies, tendons, ligaments, cartilage, or bone. Other organ systems that can cause chest pain include the respiratory, cardiovascular, gastrointestinal (GI) and nervous systems. Although the differential diagnosis of chest pain is exhaustive, chest pain in children is least likely to be cardiac in origin.

Chest pain is found equally in male and female patients, with an average age of presentation of 13 years. Children younger than 12 years are more likely to have a cardiorespiratory cause of their chest pain compared with children older than 12 years, who are more likely to have a psychogenic cause. Patients diagnosed with psychogenic chest pain or costochondritis are more likely to be female.

All complaints of chest pain should be taken seriously, but chest pain in the pediatric population is rarely associated with life-threatening disease. Chest pain persisting longer than several months is unlikely to be related to serious organic etiology. Pain that is constant or frequently occurring without completely subsiding typically is more worrisome than brief, infrequently occurring episodes of pain.

It may be helpful to understand how the patient and the parents perceive the chest pain. Simply asking the child or adolescent what he or she thinks is causing the pain may help to discover the cause.

Idiopathic is the most frequently encountered diagnosis for chest pain in pediatrics, and the pain is commonly chronic. When the history is unremarkable for serious pathology and the physical examination is normal, further testing generally is not necessary. Several studies have shown that without a specific indication, routine tests were of no benefit in determining the cause of the chest pain.

Causes of Chest Pain

Cardiac

- Angina/coronary artery disease
- Aortic or subaortic stenosis
- Arrhythmias
- Cardiomyopathy
- Coarctation of the aorta

- Cocaine ingestion
- Dissecting aortic aneurysm (in Marfan syndrome)
- Eisenmenger syndrome
- Endocarditis
- Hypertrophic cardiomyopathy
- Kawasaki disease
- Mitral valve prolapse
- Myocarditis
- Pericardial neoplasm
- Pericarditis
- Postpericardiotomy syndrome
- Rheumatic fever
- Structural abnormalities
- Supraventricular tachycardia
- Sympathomimetic ingestion
- Takayasu arteritis
- Vasospasm
- Ventricular tachycardia

Gastrointestinal

- Achalasia
- Cholecystitis
- Esophageal foreign body
- Esophageal rupture (Boerhaave syndrome)
- Esophageal spasm
- Esophagitis
- Gastritis
- Gastroesophageal reflux
- Hiatal hernia
- Mallory-Weiss tear
- Pancreatitis
- Peptic ulcer disease
- Perihepatitis (Fitz-Hugh-Curtis syndrome)
- Subdiaphragmatic abscess
- Zollinger-Ellison syndrome

Idiopathic

Musculoskeletal

- Ankylosing spondylitis
- Costochondritis
- Discitis
- Exercise
- Fibrositis
- Herniated disc
- Herpes zoster
- Metastatic disease
- Myositis
- Osteomyelitis
- Overuse injury (strain, bursitis)
- Pleurodynia
- Precordial catch syndrome
- Sickle cell vaso-occlusive crisis
- Slipping rib syndrome
- Spondylolisthesis
- Spondylolysis
- Thoracic outlet syndrome
- Transverse myelitis
- Trauma (including abuse)
- Tumor

Other

- Breast-related causes (adenocarcinoma, fibrocystic disease, gynecomastia, mastitis, thelarche)
- Castleman disease (lymph node neoplasm)
- Cigarette smoking
- Connective tissue disorders
- Cystic fibrosis
- Diabetes mellitus
- Echinococcosis
- Ehlers-Danlos syndrome
- Homocysteinuria
- Hypercoagulable syndromes
- Hyperthyroidism
- Marfan syndrome

- Mediastinal tumors
- Mediterranean fever
- Neurofibromatosis
- Spinal cord meningioma
- Spinal cord or nerve root compression

Psychiatric

- Anxiety
- Bulimia nervosa
- Depression
- Hyperventilation syndrome
- Munchausen syndrome
- Panic attacks
- Somotoform disorder
- Stress

Pulmonary

- Asthma
- Bronchiectasis
- Chronic cough
- Embolism
- Foreign body
- Infarction (sickle cell anemia)
- Pleural effusion
- Pleurisy
- Pneumonia
- Pneumomediastinum
- Pneumothorax
- Pulmonary hypertension
- Tumor

Key Historical Features

✓ Quality of pain
✓ Intensity of pain
✓ Location of pain
✓ Frequency
✓ Duration

- ✓ Radiation
- ✓ Length of time that chest pain has been present
- ✓ Relationships to exercise, eating, body position, or trauma
- ✓ Exacerbating and relieving factors
- ✓ Constitutional symptoms
  - Fever
  - Weight loss
  - Fatigue
  - Night sweats
- ✓ Cardiac symptoms
  - Palpitations
  - Racing heart
  - Dizziness
  - Syncope
- ✓ Respiratory symptoms
  - Cough
  - Shortness of breath
  - Wheezing
- ✓ Gastrointestinal symptoms
  - Nausea
  - Vomiting
  - Dysphagia
  - Heartburn
- ✓ Complete review of systems
- ✓ Past medical history, especially cardiac disease
- ✓ Past surgical history, especially heart surgery
- ✓ Medications
- ✓ Family history, especially cardiac disease or sudden death
- ✓ Social history
  - Recent stressors at home or at school
  - Family dynamics
  - Alcohol use
  - Tobacco use
  - Drug use
  - Type of work and play (specific sports activities)
  - Change in school performance

Key Physical Findings

✓   Vital signs, including blood pressure

✓   General physical examination

✓   Note interaction between the child and parent

✓   Examination of the chest for signs of injury and symmetry

✓   Palpation of the entire thoracic cage for tenderness

✓   Palpation of the precordium for signs of cardiac disease

✓   Cardiac examination for abnormal heart sounds or murmurs

✓   Pulmonary examination for evidence of accessory muscle use, infection, effusion, or bronchospasm

✓   Maneuvers to elicit the pain, such as twisting at the torso, raising the arms over the head, pushing and pulling against resistance, and deep inhalation

✓   Abdominal examination for tenderness and organ size

✓   Back examination

✓   Femoral pulses

✓   Extremity examination for temperature, cyanosis, clubbing, and edema

✓   Evaluation of the patient's psychological state

Suggested Work-Up

A thorough history and physical examination are usually all that are necessary in excluding the rare, life-threatening causes of chest pain. Laboratory testing is usually nondiagnostic, costly, and burdensome to patients. Laboratory testing is therefore most commonly unnecessary for appropriately diagnosing and treating chest pain in children. The following list is provided only as a guide to the tests that are available in diagnosing chest pain:

Cardiac

- Cardiac catheterization
- Chest radiograph
- Dobutamine stress test
- Echocardiogram
- Electrocardiogram (ECG)
- Endomyocardial biopsy with polymerase chain reaction analysis
- Exercise stress test
- Holter monitor

- Lipid profile
- Pericardiocentesis
- Thallium scan
- Serum creatinine kinase with MB fraction
- Serum troponin

Gastrointestinal

- Abdominal sonography
- Esophageal manometry
- Gastric lavage
- pH probe
- Serum amylase and lipase
- Serum gastrin level
- Serum liver function tests
- Stool guaiac testing
- Upper endoscopy
- Upper GI series

Miscellaneous

- Antinuclear antibodies
- Breast biopsy
- Breast sonography
- Coagulation studies
- Complete blood cell (CBC) count
- Cultures (blood, sputum, pericardial fluid)
- Erythrocyte sedimentation rate
- Glycosylated hemoglobin A_{1C}
- Hemoglobin electrophoresis
- Psychological testing
- Serum complement levels
- Thyroid function tests
- Toxicology screen (urine and serum)
- Tuberculosis skin test (Purified protein derivative)
- Viral or bacterial antibody titers

Musculoskeletal

- Creatine kinase with MM fraction (muscle subunits)
- Computed tomography (CT) scan of spine
- Magnetic resonance imaging (MRI) of spine

- Nuclear bone scan
- Skeletal radiographs

Pulmonary

- Bronchoscopy
- Chest radiograph
- Chloride sweat test
- CT scan of the chest
- MRI of the chest
- Pulmonary function testing with and without methacholine challenge
- Ventilation perfusion scan

References

1. Bernstein D. Evaluation of the cardiovascular system. In: Behrman RE, Kliegman RM, Jenson HB, eds. *Nelson Textbook of Pediatrics*, 17th ed. Philadelphia: WB Saunders; 2004: 1980–1981.
2. Cava JR, Sayger PL. Chest pain in children and adolescents. *Pediatr Clin North Am* 2004;51:1553–1568.
3. Driscoll DJ, Glicklich LB, Gallen WJ. Chest pain in children: a prospective study. *Pediatrics* 1976;57:648–651.
4. Kocis KC. Chest pain in pediatrics. *Pediatr Clin North Am* 1999;46:189–203.
5. Pantell RH, Goodman BW. Adolescent chest pain: a prospective study. *Pediatrics* 1983;71:881–887.
6. Selbst SM. Chest pain in children. *Pediatrics* 1985;75:1068–1070.
7. Selbst SM, Ruddy RM, Clark BJ, Henretig FM, Santulli T. Pediatric chest pain: a prospective study. *Pediatrics* 1988;82:319–323.
8. Selbt SM, Ruddy R, Clark BJ. Chest pain in children: follow-up of patients previously reported. *Clin Pediatr* 1990;29:373–377.

Theodore X. O'Connell

Chronic cough, defined as daily cough for more than 3 to 4 weeks, is a common symptom in childhood. One study found that healthy children (mean age, 10 years) have, on average, 10 cough episodes per 24 hours, mostly during the daytime. This number increases during respiratory infections, which may occur five to eight times per year in healthy children. Adding to the difficulty in treating cough, several studies have shown that the parental reporting of cough does not correlate well with the frequency, duration, or intensity of the actual cough.

In children, upper and lower respiratory tract infections, asthma, and gastroesophageal reflux disease (GERD) have been considered the most common causes of chronic cough. In older children, cough-variant asthma, sinusitis, and psychogenic cough increase in frequency. Sinusitis, tuberculosis, pertussis, and cystic fibrosis are other causes of chronic cough that should be considered. Foreign-body aspiration should be considered in younger children. Recurrent infections may indicate an underlying immunologic disorder. Rare causes that may present early in life include vascular rings, tracheoesophageal fistulas, and primary ciliary dyskinesia.

The 1998 American College of Chest Physicians guidelines advocate that "the approach to managing chronic cough in children is similar to the approach in adults." However, a subsequent study found that protracted bacterial bronchitis was the most common diagnosis in children, in contrast to adults, in whom asthma, postnasal drip syndrome, and GERD are the most common diagnoses. In fact, these adult diagnoses were found to be relatively uncommon in children. Because some controversy exists regarding the best algorithmic approach to the child with chronic cough, we provide two algorithms (Figures 10-1 and 10-2). The history and physical examination should provide significant guidance when using these algorithms. At some points in the algorithms, an empiric trial of therapy may be considered before additional testing is performed.

Up to 10% of preschool and early school-aged children have chronic cough without wheeze at some time, and parental smoking is associated with an increased prevalence of chronic cough. Fortunately, chronic cough has a favorable prognosis, with improvement being the rule in the majority of children who have chronic cough. Nonetheless, chronic cough may be the result of a serious underlying lung condition. Warning signs for serious underlying lung disease include the following:

1. Neonatal onset of the cough, which may represent a congenital defect, a problem with ciliary function (such as cystic fibrosis or primary cilial abnormality), an anatomic lesion in the airways, or a chronic viral pneumonia acquired in utero or during the perinatal period

2. Chronic moist or purulent cough
3. Cough that began and persisted after a choking episode, which may be the result of foreign body aspiration
4. Cough that occurs during or after feeding, which suggests gastroesophageal reflux or aspiration during feeding
5. General ill health with failure to thrive

Medications Associated with Chronic Cough

- Angiotensin-converting enzyme (ACE) inhibitors
- β-blockers

Causes of Chronic Cough

Aspiration

Asthma

Chronic bronchitis

Congenital abnormality

- α-1 antitrypsin deficiency
- Coarctation of the aorta
- Cysts
- Hemangioma
- Laryngeal cleft
- Mediastinal mass
- Primary ciliary dyskinesia
- Pulmonary sling
- Tracheobronchomalacia
- Tracheoesophageal fistulas
- Vascular rings

Cough-variant asthma

Cystic fibrosis

Foreign body

GERD

Immune deficiencies, especially human immunodeficiency virus (HIV) infection

Kartagener's syndrome

Post-infectious cough

Postnasal drip

Psychogenic cough

Sinusitis

Upper and lower respiratory tract infections

- *Chlamydia*
- Cytomegalovirus
- *Haemophilus influenzae*
- Mycoplasma
- Parapertussis
- Pertussis
- *Pneumocystis carinii*
- *Streptococcus pneumoniae*
- Tuberculosis
- *Ureaplasma urealytica*
- Viral

Key Historical Features

✓ Fever

✓ Severity and time course of the cough

✓ Sputum production

✓ Hemoptysis

✓ Diurnal variability

✓ Relationship of cough to meals

✓ Relationship of cough to exercise

✓ Possibility of foreign body aspiration

✓ Habitual vomiting

✓ Symptoms of asthma or known asthma triggers

✓ Heartburn or regurgitation

✓ Symptoms of postnasal drip (throat clearing, nasal discharge, excessive phlegm production)

✓ Exacerbating factors

✓ Possible allergies

✓ Purulent sputum

✓ Night sweats

✓ Weight loss

✓ Risk of contact with tuberculosis or HIV

✓ Medical history

✓ Vaccination status

✓ Medications, especially ACE-inhibitor

✓ Tobacco use

✓ Smoking behavior of parents

✓ Environmental exposures

Key Physical Findings

✓ Vital signs

✓ Height and weight measurements

✓ Head and neck examination for lymphadenopathy, evidence of allergies, sinus infection, foreign body, or poor dental hygiene

✓ Cardiac examination for evidence of left ventricular failure

✓ Pulmonary examination for any abnormal breath sounds

✓ Chest examination for a barrel-shaped chest

✓ Extremity examination for cyanosis or clubbing

✓ Skin examination for evidence of atopic disease

Suggested Work-Up

Chest radiographs	To evaluate for infiltrates, atelectasis, congenital abnormalities, radio-opaque foreign bodies, or cardiomegaly
Complete blood cell count (CBC)	To evaluate for infection or eosinophilia
Purified protein derivative (PPD)	To evaluate for tuberculosis, especially if risk factors for exposure are present

Additional Work-Up

High-resolution chest CT	May reveal bronchiectasis that is not seen on plain radiography
Sputum gram stain, cultures, and serology (e.g., *Bordetella pertussis*, *Chlamydia* spp., cytomegalovirus)	To evaluate for infection, especially if there are fevers or purulent sputum

Adenosine 5'-monophosphate bronchial challenge	To differentiate asthma from other chronic pulmonary diseases of childhood
Immunoglobulins and subclasses	To evaluate for immunologic disease
Pulmonary function tests	To evaluate for reversible obstruction
Bronchoscopy	If there is suspicion of foreign-body aspiration or congenital anomalies. Also may provide specimens from the lower airways for culture and microscopy.
Barium swallow with 24-hour esophageal pH monitoring	If reflux is suspected. Alternatively, an empiric trial of therapy may be considered.
Sinus radiographs or computed tomography (CT) scan	If sinusitis is suspected. Alternatively, an empiric trial of therapy may be considered.
Chloride sweat test	Should be performed in children with chronic cough and failure to thrive and in any child with a chronic productive cough to evaluate for cystic fibrosis
Ciliary function studies	Performed at specialized centers to evaluate for primary ciliary dyskinesia
HIV test	If risk factors for HIV exposure are present

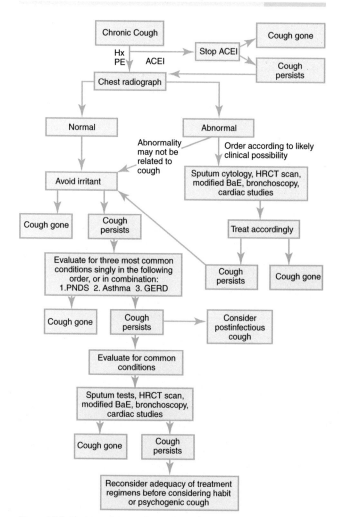

Figure 10-1. Sequential approach to the evaluation of chronic cough in the immunocompetent adult.

(From Irwin RS, et al. Managing cough as a defense mechanism and as a symptom: a consensus panel report of the American College of Chest Physicians. *Chest* 1998;114(2 suppl managing):166S.)

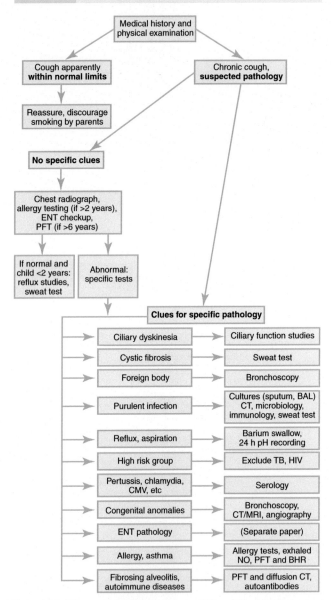

Figure 10-2. Diagnostic algorithm for use in children with chronic cough. (From de Jongste JC, Shields MD. Chronic cough in children. *Thorax* 2003;58:998–1003, with permission.)

References

1. Archer LNJ, Simpson H. Night cough counts and diary card scores in asthma. *Arch Dis Child* 1998;60:473–474.
2. de Jongste JC, Shields MD. Chronic cough in children. *Thorax* 2003;58:998–1003.
3. Falconer A, Oldman C, Helms P. Poor agreement between reported and recorded nocturnal cough in asthma. *Pediatr Pulmonol* 1993;15:209–211.
4. Holmes RL, Fadded CT. Evaluation of the patient with chronic cough. *Am Fam Physician* 2004;69:2159–2166.
5. Irwin RS, et al. Managing cough as a defense mechanism and as a symptom: a consensus panel report of the American College of Chest Physicians. *Chest* 1998;114(2 suppl managing):166S.
6. Kamei RK. Chronic cough in children. *Pediatr Clin North Am* 1991;38:593–605.
7. Marchant JM, et al. Evaluation and outcome of young children with chronic cough. *Chest* 2006;129:1132–1141.
8. Munyard P, Bush A. How much coughing is normal? *Arch Dis Child* 1996;74:531–534.

Theodore X. O'Connell

The term *constipation* has different meanings to different people. Constipation may be defined as a delay or difficulty in defecation, present for 2 or more weeks, sufficient to cause significant distress to the patient. It must be considered that there is a wide variability in normal defecation frequency in young children. As children age, the daily number of stools decreases from a mean of 2.2 in infants younger than 1 year to a mean of 1.4 in 1- to 3-year-old children. *Encopresis,* the involuntary leakage of feces into the undergarments, may be an indication of constipation.

Constipation frequently begins with feeding transitions, such as the change from breast milk to formula, or from strained foods to table foods. The transition to a daycare setting or an all-day school may also be a contributing factor to constipation. The passage of a hard or large stool may cause a painful anal fissure, which may create a fear of painful defecation. This may result in a cycle of avoiding bowel movements and progress to stool retention. As the child avoids defecating, the rectum eventually stretches to accommodate the retained fecal mass, and the propulsive power of the rectum is diminished.

In children younger than one year of age, the possibility of Hirschsprung disease must be considered. Approximately 40% of children with functional constipation develop symptoms during the first year of life. Functional constipation is the diagnosis in more than 95% of cases of constipation in children older than 1 year. The passage of infrequent, large-caliber stools is highly suggestive of functional constipation. The Rome III criteria for functional constipation are outlined below. Note that the criteria are different depending whether the child is older or younger than 4 years of age (Table 11-1).

Although the differential diagnosis of constipation is extensive, the diagnosis frequently can be made on the basis of a history and physical examination. A 1-week symptom and diet history may be helpful in determining the cause of childhood constipation. Red flag signs and symptoms include the following:

✓ Passage of meconium more than 48 hours after delivery, small-caliber stools, failure to thrive, fever, bilious vomiting, bloody diarrhea, tight anal sphincter, and empty rectum with palpable abdominal fecal mass (all are suggestive of Hirschsprung disease)

✓ Delayed growth

✓ Polyuria and polydipsia

✓ Failure to thrive, fever, rash, and recurrent pneumonia (suggestive of cystic fibrosis)

For infants up to 4 years of age, at least 2 of the following criteria must be present for 1 month:	For a child with a developmental age of at least 4 years, 2 or more of the following criteria must be present at least once per week for at least 2 months with insufficient criteria for the diagnosis of irritable bowel syndrome (IBS):
1. Two or fewer defecations per week 2. At least 1 episode per week of incontinence after the acquisition of toileting skills 3. History of excessive stool retention 4. History of painful or hard bowel movements 5. Presence of a large fecal mass in the rectum 6. History of large-diameter stools that may obstruct the toilet	1. Two or fewer defecations in the toilet per week 2. At least 1 episode of fecal incontinence per week 3. History of retentive posturing or excessive volitional stool retention 4. History of painful or hard bowel movements 5. Presence of a large fecal mass in the rectum 6. History of large diameter stools that may obstruct the toilet

Table 11-1. Rome III Criteria for Functional Constipation

✓   Urinary incontinence

✓   Absent cremasteric reflex; absence of anal wink; a decrease in lower extremity reflexes or muscular tone; or the presence of a pilonidal dimple, pigment changes, or hair tuft in the sacrococcygeal area (suggestive of spinal cord abnormalities)

✓   Abnormal anal position or appearance on physical examination

In the absence of red flag symptoms, no testing or subspecialist consultation is needed before treatment is initiated.

Medications Associated with Constipation

- Antacids
- Anticholinergics
- Antidepressants
- Bismuth
- Laxatives
- Opiates
- Phenobarbital
- Sympathomimetics

Causes of Constipation

Connective tissue disorders

- Scleroderma
- Systemic lupus erythematosus

Endocrine causes

- Diabetes insipidus

- Diabetes mellitus
- Pregnancy

Functional causes

- Dehydration
- Excessive cow's milk intake
- Inadequate dietary fiber
- Malnutrition
- Motility disturbance (slow transit)
- Sexual abuse
- Stool withholding

Genetic and immunologic causes

- Celiac disease
- Cystic fibrosis
- Inflammatory bowel disease
- Neurofibromatosis

Medications

Metabolic causes

- Heavy metal poisoning
- Hypercalcemia
- Hyperparathyroidism
- Hypokalemia
- Hypothyroidism
- Uremia

Neurogenic causes

- Cerebral palsy
- Developmental delay
- Hypotonia from Down syndrome or prune-belly syndrome
- Myelomeningocele
- Spina bifida
- Spinal tumors
- Tethered cord

Neuromuscular causes

- Chagas' disease
- Hirschsprung's disease (aganglionosis)
- Infant botulism
- Pseudo-obstruction syndrome

Structural abnormalities

- Anal fissure
- Anal stenosis
- Anteriorly displaced anus
- Colonic stricture (primary or secondary)
- Imperforate anus
- Pelvic mass (sacral teratoma)

Key Historical Features

✓ Time of onset of the problem

✓ Frequency of the stool

✓ Consistency of the stool

✓ Caliber of the stool

✓ Volume of the stool

✓ Episodes of pain with defecation

✓ Abdominal pain

✓ Blood on the stool or the toilet paper

✓ Fecal incontinence

✓ Stool withholding behavior

✓ Urinary problems

✓ Neurologic deficits

✓ Time after birth of the first bowel movement

✓ Growth history

✓ Past medical history

✓ Past surgical history

✓ Medications

✓ Family history

✓ Review of systems, including fever, fatigue, cold intolerance, polyuria, polydipsia, diarrhea, rash, abdominal distention, bilious vomiting

Key Physical Findings

✓ Vital signs

✓ Growth parameters

✓ General appearance

✓ Head and neck examination

✓ Cardiopulmonary examination

✓ Abdominal examination to evaluate for a fecal mass in the suprapubic area and for distention or organomegaly

✓ Back and spine examination for pigment abnormalities or hair tufts in the sacrococcygeal area

✓ Examination of the perineum and anus

✓ Genital examination for cremasteric reflex

✓ Digital rectal examination should be performed to assess rectal tone and determine the presence of rectal distention or impaction

✓ Neurologic examination for tone, strength, and deep tendon reflexes

Suggested Work-Up

Fecal occult blood testing	Recommended in all infants with constipation and in children of any age who have abdominal pain, failure to thrive, intermittent diarrhea, or a family history of colon cancer or colon polyps
Plain-film radiography of the abdomen	May be helpful to assess the presence of a fecal mass in a child who is not cooperative with abdominal or rectal examination

Additional Work-Up

Thyroid function tests	If thyroid dysfunction is suspected
Serum electrolytes, calcium, and magnesium	If a metabolic disorder is suspected
Lead level	If lead toxicity is suspected
Barium enema	To evaluate for anatomic abnormalities, Hirschsprung disease or colonic strictures
Anorectal manometry	To evaluate the rectoanal inhibitory reflex and to evaluate for Hirschsprung disease
Suction rectal biopsy	To establish a tissue diagnosis of Hirschsprung disease

Magnetic resonance imaging (MRI) of the lumbosacral spine	If a spinal problem such as tethered cord, sacral agenesis, or tumor is suspected
Endomesial and tissue transglutaminase antibodies	If celiac disease is suspected on the basis of symptoms developing after wheat is introduced into the diet
Transit study	May be considered in a child with infrequent bowel movements and no signs of constipation to evaluate transit time

References

1. Abi-Hanna A, Lake AM. Constipation and encopresis in childhood. *Pediatr Rev* 1998; 19:23–30.
2. Arce DA, Ermocilla CA, Costa H. Evaluation of constipation. *Am Fam Physician* 2002;65:2283–2290.
3. Baker SS, et al. Constipation in infants and children: evaluation and treatment. A medical position statement of the North American Society for Pediatric Gastroenterology and Nutrition. *J Pediatr Gastroenterol Nutr* 1999;29:612–626.
4. Biggs WS, Dery WH. Evaluation and treatment of constipation in infants and children. *Am Fam Physician* 2006;73:469–477.
5. Hyman PE, et al. Childhood functional gastrointestinal disorders: neonate/toddler. *Gastroenterology* 2006;130:1519–1526.
6. Rasquin A, et al. Childhood functional gastrointestinal disorders: child/adolescent. *Gastroenterology* 2006;130:1527–1537.
7. Reuchlin-Vrocklage LM, Bierma-Zeinstra S, Benninga MA, Berger MY. Diagnostic value of abdominal radiography in constipated children. *Arch Pediatr Adolesc Med* 2005;159: 671–678.

Theodore X. O'Connell

Cyanosis is a blue to dusky hue which may be seen in the newborn. Bruising or ecchymosis may look like cyanosis and is differentiated by applying pressure over the skin, which will blanch with cyanosis but not with ecchymosis. *Central cyanosis* involves the entire body, including the mucous membranes and tongue. *Peripheral cyanosis, or acrocyanosis,* is limited to the extremities.

Arterial blood oxygen content is normal in peripheral cyanosis, whereas arterial blood oxygen content is decreased in central cyanosis. Although peripheral cyanosis may be seen with exposure to the cold, it may also be the presenting sign of serious conditions such as sepsis, hypoglycemia, or hypoplastic left-sided heart syndrome. Therefore, peripheral cyanosis should not be ignored unless other conditions have been ruled out.

In addition to central and peripheral cyanosis, cyanosis has several other patterns. In *differential cyanosis,* the upper part of the body remains pink while the lower part of the body remains cyanotic. This pattern is seen in conditions in which there is right-to-left shunt from the pulmonary artery to the descending aorta through a patent ductus arteriosus (PDA). In *reverse differential cyanosis,* the upper part of the body remains cyanotic, whereas the lower part remains pink. Reverse differential cyanosis may occur in transposition of the great vessels with pulmonary hypertension and shunt through a PDA and total anomalous pulmonary venous return above the diaphragm with shunt through a PDA. *Harlequin condition* is a unique phenomenon in which one quadrant or one half of the body may become cyanotic while the rest of the body remains pink. This condition is thought to result from vasomotor instability.

During the assessment of cyanosis in the newborn, it is important to identify the cause of cyanosis on a physiologic basis. The two most common causes of cyanosis are **cardiac** and **pulmonary** conditions. Cyanosis also may result from abnormalities in the oxygen carrying states of the hemoglobin, metabolic causes, central nervous system (CNS) conditions, and sepsis. Other causes are outlined below.

Because most causes for cyanosis are attributable to cardiopulmonary problems, it is important to differentiate between cardiac and pulmonary causes. The hyperoxia test, described below, can help differentiate between cardiac and noncardiac causes. Respiratory disease is more likely in newborns who are tachypneic and using accessory muscles of respiration.

Cyanotic congenital heart defects that are not detected in the newborn nursery will present during the first 2 to 3 weeks of life when the ductus arteriosus closes. Echocardiogram is indicated in these patients.

Causes of Cyanosis

Cardiac Causes

- Coarctation of the aorta
- Double-outlet right ventricle
- Ebstein's anomaly
- Interrupted aortic arch
- Hypoplastic left heart syndrome
- Left-to-right shunt with pulmonary edema
- Low cardiac output states
- Pulmonary atresia
- Pulmonary stenosis
- Single ventricle states
- Tetralogy of Fallot (TOF)
- Total anomalous pulmonary venous return (TAPVR)
- Transposition of the great arteries (TGA)
- Tricuspid atresia
- Truncus arteriosus

Pulmonary Causes

- Aspiration (meconium, blood, amniotic fluid, mucus, or milk)
- Choanal atresia
- Congenital cystic adenomatoid malformation (CCAM)
- Congenital diaphragmatic hernia (CDH)
- Hyaline membrane disease (HMD)
- Laryngeal web
- Lobar emphysema
- Persistent pulmonary hypertension of the newborn (PPHN)
- Pierre Robin syndrome
- Pleural effusion
- Pneumomediastinum
- Pneumonia
- Pneumothorax
- Pulmonary edema
- Pulmonary hemorrhage
- Pulmonary hypoplasia
- Pulmonary lymphangiectasia
- Pulmonary sequestration

- Respiratory distress syndrome
- Tracheoesophageal fistula (TEF)

CNS Causes

- Apnea
- Asphyxia
- Cerebral edema
- Hemorrhage
- Hypoventilation
- Infection
- Seizures
- Vocal cord paralysis or paresis

Miscellaneous Causes

- Abdominal distension
- Gastroesophageal reflux
- Hemoglobin M
- Hypocalcemia
- Hypoglycemia
- Hypomagnesemia
- Hypothermia
- Metabolic acidosis
- Methemoglobinemia
- Polycythemia
- Sepsis
- Sulfhemoglobinemia

Key Historical Features

Onset of Cyanosis

✓ Onset at birth may result from transient tachypnea of the newborn (TTN), respiratory distress syndrome, pneumothorax, meconium aspiration syndrome, CDH, or CCAM

✓ Onset several hours after birth may be related to cyanotic congenital heart disease, postnatal aspiration syndromes, or TEF

Maternal History

✓ Maternal diabetes increases the risk of TTN, HMD, and hypoglycemia

✓ Asthma increases risk of TTN

✓ Narcotic use may lead to narcotic withdrawal, often 36 to 48 hours after birth

✓ Pregnancy-induced hypertension increases risk of polycythemia and hypoglycemia

Labor and Delivery History

✓ Prolonged rupture of membranes increases the risk of sepsis and pneumonia

✓ Intrapartum fever increases the risk of infection in the newborn

✓ Narcotic analgesia or anesthesia increases the risk of newborn cyanosis

✓ Nonreassuring fetal heart-rate tracings and perinatal hypoxic depression at birth increase the risk of hypotension, metabolic acidosis, and cerebral edema in the newborn

✓ Cesarean section deliveries without labor are associated with a higher risk of TTN and persistent pulmonary hypertension

✓ Difficult vaginal delivery may cause an Erb palsy with associated phrenic nerve paralysis, leading to respiratory distress

Prenatal History That May Increase Risk of Polycythemia and Hypoglycemia

✓ Oligohydramnios may lead to pulmonary hypoplasia

✓ Polyhydramnios may be associated with TEF, neurologic conditions, or anatomic abnormalities of the gastrointestinal (GI) tract

Family History

✓ A sibling with a history of early onset invasive group B streptococcal (GBS) disease confers a higher risk of early onset GBS infection

✓ A family history of congenital heart disease increases the risk of recurrence

✓ A sibling with a history of surfactant protein B deficiency increases the risk of recurrence

Key Physical Findings

✓ Vital signs

✓ Blood pressure measurement in all four extremities

✓ Determination of whether cyanosis is peripheral or central

✓ Head and neck examination for nasal flaring: holding the bell of the stethoscope over the nostrils may help identify nasal obstruction from choanal atresia

✓ Cardiac examination for heart rate, heart sounds, and murmurs; location of the apical impulse and presence of a precordial thrill

✓ Evaluation of respirations for respiratory rate, retractions, and grunting

✓ Evaluation of the shape of the chest

✓ Pulmonary examination for equal air entry bilaterally, presence of breath sounds in all lung fields, rales, and rhonchi

✓ Abdominal examination for distension, hepatosplenomegaly, and bowel sounds

✓ Assessment of perfusion by capillary refill time

✓ Palpation of both brachial and femoral pulses with assessment of the quality and volume of the pulses

✓ Neurologic examination for hypotonia or Erb palsy

Suggested Work-Up

Pulse oximetry monitoring	If there is severe cyanosis with respiratory distress, the pulse oximeter should be placed over the right hand and a lower extremity to detect the gradient across the ductus arteriosus
Hyperoxia test	Indicated if the infant's pulse oximeter reading is less than 85% on both room air and 100% oxygen
	An arterial blood gas (ABG) is obtained on room air; the infant is placed on 100% oxygen for 10 to 15 minutes, then the ABG is repeated. If the cause of cyanosis is pulmonary, the PaO_2 should increase by 30 mm Hg. If the cause is cardiac, there should be minimal improvement in the PaO_2. The initial ABG should be obtained with co-oximetry because methemoglobinemia can also cause cyanosis
Chest radiograph	To determine the locations of the stomach, liver, and heart to evaluate for dextrocardia and situs inversus. To evaluate the size and shape of the heart; pulmonary vascular markings, lung volumes, and interstitial markings; pneumothorax, pleural effusion, infiltrates, or elevated hemidiaphragms. To evaluate the bony thoracic cage and to look for fractures of the ribs, humerus, or clavicles
Electrocardiogram (ECG)	To evaluate for arrhythmias

Echocardiogram	To evaluate for congenital cardiac lesions and pulmonary hypertension
CBC with differential count	To evaluate for polycythemia, anemia, neutropenia, leukopenia, abnormal immature-to-total neutrophil ratio, and thrombocytopenia
Blood culture	If sepsis is suspected
Spinal tap	If sepsis is suspected

Additional Work-Up

Serum electrolytes	To evaluate for electrolyte abnormalities contributing to heart block if the infant's heart rate does not increase appropriately with stimulation
Serum calcium and magnesium	Should be obtained in newborns in whom other causes are ruled out
Ultrasound	To evaluate for pleural effusion or paradoxical motion of the diaphragm
Computed tomography (CT) scan of the chest	May be helpful if the diagnosis is not clear and in detecting congenital abnormalities and tumors of the mediastinum, lungs, and heart
Upper GI contrast study	To evaluate for severe gastroesophageal reflux and esophagitis when cyanosis occurs with feeding
Metabolic screening of urine and drug screening of urine and meconium	If clinically indicated

References

1. Brousseau T, Sharieff GQ. Newborn emergencies: the first 30 days of life. *Pediatr Clin North Am* 2006;53:69–84.
2. Fuloria M, Kreiter S. The newborn examination: part I. Emergencies and common abnormalities involving the skin, head, neck, chest, and respiratory and cardiovascular systems. *Am Fam Physician* 2002;65:61–68.
3. Hashim MJ, Guillet R. Common issues in the care of sick neonates. *Am Fam Physician* 2002;66:1685–1692.
4. Sasidharan P. An approach to diagnosis and management of cyanosis and tachypnea in term infants. *Pediatr Clin North Am* 2005;51:999–1021.

Theodore X. O'Connell

The term *diarrhea* refers to an increase in the frequency, fluidity, or volume of bowel movements relative to the usual habit of an individual. The World Health Organization (WHO) defines diarrhea as the passage of three or more loose or watery stools per day. An acute diarrheal illness typically is defined as a duration of 5 days or less. Children younger than 5 years old in developing countries have three to nine diarrheal illnesses per year, whereas in North America, young children have on average two diarrheal episodes per year.

Acute viral gastroenteritis is the most common cause of acute gastroenteritis in developed countries. Of the viral agents, rotavirus is the most common. Other common causes of diarrhea are bacterial infections, systemic nongastrointestinal infection, and antibiotics. Potentially life-threatening causes of diarrhea include hemolytic uremic syndrome (HUS), intussusception, pseudomembranous colitis, toxic megacolon, and appendicitis.

In contrast to the largely viral causation of gastroenteritis in the United States, diarrhea acquired in developing countries is more frequently bacterial in origin. *Escherichia coli* (*E. coli*), the most frequently isolated pathogen, may cause diarrhea of varying types and severity. Enterotoxigenic *E. coli* usually produces a mild, self-limited illness without significant fever or systemic toxicity, although it may be severe in newborns and infants. Enteroinvasive strains of *E. coli* cause a more significant illness characterized by fever, systemic symptoms, blood and mucus in the stool, and leukocytosis. Other invasive pathogens include *Campylobacter, Shigella,* and nontyphoid *Salmonella. Aeromonas* and noncholera *Vibrio* spp. are encountered less frequently.

Dehydration is the main complication of acute diarrhea. HUS is characterized by microangiopathic hemolytic anemia, thrombocytopenia, and renal failure. HUS is strongly associated with Shiga toxin–producing *E. coli,* although other strains and bacteria have been implicated.

Causes of Acute Diarrhea

Antibiotic Administration

Bacillus cereus–preformed toxin

Food poisoning

Gastrointestinal (GI) Infection

Bacterial

- *Aeromonas*
- *Campylobacter*
- *Clostridium difficile*
- *E. coli*

- *Salmonella* (nontyphoid)
- *Shigella*
- *Vibrio* (noncholera)
- *Yersinia*

Parasites

- *Cryptosporidium parvum*
- *Cyclospora cayetanensis*
- *Entamoeba histolytica*
- *Giardia lamblia*

Viral

- Adenovirus
- Norwalk and Norwalk-like virus
- Rotavirus

HUS

Intussusception

Nongastrointestinal Infection

- Appendicitis
- Urinary tract infection (UTI)

Overfeeding

Seafood ingestion syndromes

- Ciguatera poisoning
- Scombroid poisoning

Staphylococcus aureus-preformed toxin

Toxic Megacolon

Key Historical Features

✓ Fever

✓ Duration of diarrhea

✓ Frequency of diarrhea

✓ Presence of blood in the diarrhea

✓ Abdominal pain

✓ Vomiting

✓ Fluid intake

✓ Urine output

✓ Recent antibiotic use

✓ Review of systems, especially urinary symptoms

✓   Medical history, especially immunocompromised status

✓   Surgical history

✓   Family history

✓   Recent travel

Key Physical Findings

✓   Vital signs

✓   General appearance

✓   General examination for evidence of dehydration

- Head and neck examination for dry mucous membranes and the absence of tears
- Cardiovascular examination for tachycardia
- Extremity examination for capillary refill and skin turgor

✓   Abdominal examination for bowel sounds, distension, tenderness

Suggested Work-Up

The extent of evaluation of stool specimens from a specific patient should be determined by the patient's symptoms, time to onset of disease, age of the patient, travel history, food consumed, immunologic status, and prior history of antibiotic use. In most children with watery diarrhea and no associated symptoms such as fever, abdominal pain, blood or mucus in the stools and no history of diarrheal outbreak or toxin exposure, laboratory investigation is not required.

Stool leukocyte examination	Useful in patients with moderate to severe diarrhea with any associated symptoms such as fever, abdominal pain, blood or mucus in the stools, history of diarrheal outbreak, or toxin exposure
Stool culture	If the patient is febrile and has bloody diarrhea or if the stool leukocytes are positive
Urine culture	Should be considered in febrile children under 1 year of age
Serum electrolytes	If the patient is ill-appearing or appears significantly dehydrated

Stool for *Clostridium difficile* toxin	If the patient has bloody diarrhea and has been on antibiotics in the preceding 3 to 6 months
Stool for ova and parasites	If the patient has traveled to an endemic area

Additional Work-Up

Complete blood count (CBC), chemistry panel, C-reactive protein, serum lactate dehydrogenase, urinalysis, and stool culture	If hemolytic uremic syndrome is suspected
Abdominal ultrasound	May be used if intussusception is suspected
Air contrast barium enema	If intussusception is suspected. May be therapeutic in such cases
Abdominal computed tomography (CT) scan	If an intra abdominal process such as appendicitis is suspected
Colonoscopy	May be indicated to establish the diagnosis of pseudomembranous colitis
Mucosal biopsy specimens for cytomegalovirus identification and culture	May be indicated in immunocompromised children

References

1. Fasano A. Clinical presentation of celiac disease in the pediatric population. *Gastroenterology* 2005;128:S68–S73.
2. Ramaswamy K, Jacobson K. Infectious diarrhea in children. *Gastroenterol Clin* 2001;30: 611–624.
3. Razzaq S. Hemolytic uremic syndrome: an emerging health risk. *Am Fam Physician* 2006;74:991–996.
4. Yates J. Traveler's diarrhea. *Am Fam Physician* 2005;71:2095–2100.

Theodore X. O'Connell

The term *diarrhea* refers to an increase in the frequency, fluidity, or volume of bowel movements relative to the usual habit of an individual. The World Health Organization (WHO) defines diarrhea as the passage of three or more loose or watery stools per day. Diarrhea may be considered chronic if it persists for 14 days or longer.

Gastrointestinal (GI) infection is the most common cause of chronic diarrhea in children. The major pathogens are outlined below. Protein intolerance, usually to cow's milk or soy protein, is a common cause of chronic diarrhea and usually manifests before 6 months of age. Protein intolerance may be accompanied by bloody diarrhea, anemia, and manifestations of allergy, such as eczema, hives, or asthma.

Chronic nonspecific diarrhea of childhood primarily affects children between 1 and 5 years of age. Although the parents may be concerned, children with chronic nonspecific diarrhea do not suffer from their ailment and appear healthy. The syndrome is characterized by persistent or recurrent episodes of voluminous loose stools, often with undigested food particles in the stools. Nocturnal diarrhea is absent. The pathophysiology of chronic nonspecific diarrhea remains unclear.

Overfeeding results in an osmotic diarrhea, often from the excessive intake of fluids containing sorbitol and fructose. Primary disaccharidase deficiencies are rare. However, secondary disaccharidase deficiencies occur more commonly as a result of damage to the brush-border membrane and may be associated with infection, allergies, and celiac disease. The diarrhea typically is explosive and watery and may be accompanied by bloating, flatulence, and abdominal pain.

Celiac disease is associated with villous atrophy of the proximal small intestine as a result of intolerance to gluten protein. Most children with celiac disease begin to show symptoms at 6 to 24 months of age, although symptoms can develop anytime after gluten is introduced into the diet in the form of wheat, barley, or rye. In addition to chronic diarrhea, children with celiac disease may have failure to thrive, irritability, muscle wasting, abdominal distention, and anorexia.

Cystic fibrosis may manifest as steatorrhea with malabsorption. The history may include meconium inspissation in the neonatal period, prolonged neonatal jaundice, and recurrent or chronic chest infections.

Inflammatory bowel disease usually develops in late childhood or during adolescence. Bloody diarrhea, abdominal pain, and weight loss should raise suspicion for ulcerative colitis or Crohn's disease. Both conditions may be accompanied by extraintestinal manifestations such as arthritis, intermittent fever, erythema nodosum, and pyoderma gangrenosum.

Pseudomembranous enterocolitis is infrequently diagnosed in children but may be seen following antibiotic administration. Antibiotics may also cause diarrhea as a result of bacterial overgrowth.

Endocrine causes of chronic diarrhea include hyperthyroidism, diabetes mellitus, adrenal insufficiency, and hypoparathyroidism. Functional tumors may result in chronic diarrhea by secreting hormones. These tumors are outlined below. Other less common causes of chronic diarrhea are also outlined below.

Causes of Chronic Diarrhea

Acquired monosaccharide malabsorption

Adrenal insufficiency

Anatomic lesions

- Blind loop syndrome
- Hirschsprung disease
- Intestinal pseudo-obstruction syndrome
- Lymphoma
- Lymphosarcoma
- Malrotation
- Partial small bowel obstruction
- Polyposis
- Short bowel syndrome

Antibiotics

Carbohydrate malabsorption

Celiac disease

Chronic constipation with overflow diarrhea

Chronic nonspecific diarrhea of childhood

Congenital chloride-losing diarrhea

Crohn's disease

Diabetes mellitus

Dietary

- Malnutrition
- Milk protein hypersensitivity
- Overfeeding
- Sorbitol intolerance
- Soy protein hypersensitivity

Disaccharidase deficiencies

Enterokinase deficiency

Eosinophilic gastroenteropathy

Glucoamylase deficiency

Glucose-galactose malabsorption

Hormone-secreting tumors

- APUDomas
- Carcinoid tumor
- Ganglioneuroma
- Medullary carcinoma of the thyroid
- Neuroblastoma
- Pancreatic islet cell tumor (Zollinger-Ellison syndrome)

Hyperthyroidism

Hypoparathyroidism

Immunodeficiency states

- Acquired immunodeficiency syndrome (AIDS)
- Agammaglobulinemia
- Autoimmune enteropathy
- Combined immunodeficiency
- Defective cellular immunity
- Isolated IgA deficiency

Infections

- Bacterial
  - *Campylobacter jejuni*
  - *Escherichia coli*
  - *Salmonella species*
  - *Shigella* spp.
  - *Yersinia enterocolitica*
- Parasitic
  - Cryptosporidium species
  - *Entamoeba histolytica*
  - *Giardia lamblia*
- Viral
  - Adenovirus
  - Enteroviruses
  - Norwalk virus
  - Rotavirus

Intestinal ischemia

Intestinal lymphangiectasia

Lactase deficiency

Laxative use

Liver disorders

- Biliary atresia
- Chronic hepatitis
- Primary bile acid malabsorption

Metabolic abnormalities

- Abetalipoproteinemia
- Acrodermatitis enteropathica
- Familial chloride diarrhea
- Folic acid malabsorption
- Galactosemia
- Hypobetalipoproteinemia
- Selective vitamin B_{12} malabsorption
- Sodium-hydrogen exchange defect
- Tyrosinemia
- Wolman's disease

Microvillus inclusion disease

Necrotizing enterocolitis

Pancreatic disorders

- Chronic pancreatitis
- Cystic fibrosis
- Johanson-Blizzard syndrome
- Lipase deficiency
- Shwachman-Diamond syndrome
- Trypsinogen deficiency

Pseudomembranous enterocolitis

Sucrase-isomaltase deficiency

Toxic diarrhea

Tropical sprue

Ulcerative colitis

Urinary tract infection (UTI)

Whipple disease

Key Historical Features

✓   Age of onset

✓   Duration of diarrhea

✓   Frequency of diarrhea

- ✓ Presence of blood in the diarrhea
- ✓ Appearance of the stools
- ✓ Abdominal pain
- ✓ Vomiting
- ✓ Fluid intake
- ✓ Urine output
- ✓ Recent antibiotic use
- ✓ Exposure to infectious agents
- ✓ Associated symptoms
  - Fever
  - Weight loss
  - Arthritis
  - Rash or skin lesions
  - Chest infections
  - Heat intolerance or nervousness
- ✓ Review of systems, especially urinary symptoms
- ✓ Dietary history and relationship of diarrhea to diet
- ✓ Medical history, especially immunocompromised status
- ✓ Surgical history
- ✓ Family history especially celiac disease, cystic fibrosis, inflammatory bowel disease
- ✓ Recent travel

Key Physical Findings

- ✓ Vital signs
- ✓ Weight, height, and head circumference
- ✓ General appearance
- ✓ General examination for evidence of dehydration
- ✓ Head and neck examination for nasal polyps or iritis
- ✓ Abdominal examination for bowel sounds, distension, tenderness
- ✓ Rectal examination for prolapse, fissure, fistula, or abscess
- ✓ Extremity examination for digital clubbing, arthritis, tremor, or edema
- ✓ Skin examination for eczematous dermatitis, dermatitis herpetiformis, erythema nodosum, or pyoderma gangrenosum

Suggested Work-Up

Stool analysis for the following:

pH and reducing substances	The presence of reducing substances with a pH less than 6 suggests carbohydrate malabsorption
Occult blood	To evaluate for bleeding
Fatty acid crystals	Suggests a mucosal problem such as celiac disease
Fat globules	The presence of fat globules in an older child suggests steatorrhea but may be normal in the first few months of life
Microscopic exam for red blood cells (RBCs) and white blood cells (WBCs)	Neutrophils and RBCs may suggest infection or inflammatory bowel disease Eosinophils suggest parasitic infestation or protein intolerance
Microscopic exam for ova and parasites	To evaluate for parasite infection
Stool culture	To evaluate for infectious etiologies
Complete blood cell count (CBC)	To evaluate for infection, neutropenia, or eosinophilia. May also reveal microcytic or macrocytic anemia
Erythrocyte sedimentation rate	To evaluate for infection or inflammatory bowel disease
Serum electrolytes	To evaluate for electrolyte disturbance
Serum protein and albumin levels	To evaluate for malnutrition (proportional decrease) or protein-losing enteropathy (greater loss of albumin)
Serum carotene level	To evaluate for fat malabsorption

Additional Work-Up

Endomysial and tissue transglutaminase antibodies	If celiac disease is suspected
Giardia stool antigen	If giardiasis is suspected
Serum immunoglobulins	If immunodeficiency is suspected
HIV test	If HIV infection is suspected
Hydrogen breath test	If carbohydrate malabsorption is suspected
72-hour fecal fat test	If fat malabsorption is suspected
Sweat chloride test	If cystic fibrosis is suspected
Upper GI series with small-bowel follow-through	If Crohn's disease or anatomic abnormalities are suspected
Barium enema	If Hirschsprung's disease or inflammatory bowel disease is suspected
Sigmoidoscopy	If inflammatory bowel disease or pseudomembranous colitis is suspected
Jejunal biopsy	To confirm the presence of celiac disease

References

1. Branski D, Lerner A, Lebenthal E. Chronic diarrhea and malabsorption. *Pediatr Clin North Am* 1996;43:307–328.
2. Fasano A. Clinical presentation of celiac disease in the pediatric population. *Gastroenterology* 2005;128:S68–S73.
3. Hyman PE, Milla PJ, Benninga MA, Davidson GP, Fleisher DF, Taminiau J. et al. Childhood functional gastrointestinal disorders: neonate/toddler. *Gastroenterology* 2006;130: 1519–1526.
4. Kneepkens CMF, Hoekstra JH. Chronic nonspecific diarrhea of childhood: pathophysiology and management. *Pediatr Clin North Am* 1996;43:375–390.
5. Leung AKC, Robson WLM. Evaluating the child with chronic diarrhea. *Am Fam Physician* 1996;53:635–643.

Theodore X. O'Connell

Encopresis refers to the involuntary loss of formed, semiformed, or liquid stool into the child's underwear after the child has reached the age of 4 years. Encopresis most commonly occurs in the presence of functional constipation, which is constipation not due to organic and anatomic causes or intake of medication. Encopresis also may occur when fecal retention is not a primary etiologic component. Various terms have been used to describe this problem, including functional encopresis, primary nonretentive encopresis, and stool toileting refusal. These children may be further divided into at least four subgroups: (1) those who fail to obtain initial bowel training, (2) those who exhibit toilet "phobia," (3) those who use soiling to manipulate their environment, and (4) those who have irritable bowel syndrome (IBS). In these cases, constipation is not contributory but rather represents the child refusing the toilet-training process.

Encopresis affects 1% to 3% of children. Of encopresis cases, 80% to 95% involve fecal constipation and retention, with the remainder representing refusal of the toilet training process as described above. Stool retention results when stool expulsion has not occurred for several days. If stool retention persists, then formed, soft, or semiliquid stools leak to the outside around the accumulated firm stool mass. When stool retention remains untreated for a prolonged period, the rectum becomes stretched and a megarectum develops. The intervals between bowel movements then become increasingly longer, and the rectum becomes so large that the stored stool may be palpated as an abdominal mass that can reach the level of the umbilicus.

In general, the constipated school-age child is brought to medical attention because of encopresis, often of many years' duration, or because of abdominal pain. Encopresis often occurs in the afternoon, when the child is in an upright position, especially during exercise.

A careful history and physical examination allow the physician to make a decision regarding requirements for blood tests, radiographic studies, anorectal manometric studies, or rectal biopsy. An important part of the evaluation is assessment of fecal retention. A positive rectal examination is sufficient to document fecal retention. A negative rectal examination or a child's refusal to cooperate with rectal examination requires plain abdominal films to confirm the presence of fecal retention. The evaluation of constipation is described in detail in another chapter.

Suggested Work-Up

Most cases of encopresis are of the retentive type and are associated with chronic constipation. For the child who refuses the toilet-training process, an assessment of the child's physical, cognitive, and emotional maturity is appropriate. If the child possesses readiness skills, then behavior management and toilet training strategies should be discussed with the parents.

References

1. Boris NW, Dalton R. In: Behrman RE, Kliegman RM, Jenson HB, eds. *Nelson Textbook of Pediatrics*, 17th ed. Philadelphia: WB Saunders, 2004.
2. Kuhn BR, Marcus BA, Pitner SL. Treatment guidelines for primary nonretentive encopresis and stool toileting refusal. *Am Fam Physician* 1999;59:2171–2178.
3. Loening-Baucke V. Encopresis and soiling. *Pediatr Clin North Am* 1996;43:279–298.

Jonathan M. Wong and Timothy J. Horita

Failure to thrive (FTT) is a descriptive term and not a specific diagnosis. FTT is best defined as inadequate physical growth diagnosed by observation of growth over time using a standard growth chart. Most practitioners diagnose FTT when a child's weight for age falls below the fifth percentile of the standard National Center for Health Statistics (NCHS) growth chart or if it crosses two major percentile lines.

Average birth weight for a term infant is 3.3 kg (7.27 lb). Weight declines as much as 10% in the first few days of life, probably as a result of loss of excess fluid. Birth weight should be regained within 2 weeks after birth. Breast-fed infants tend to regain birth weight a little later than bottle-fed infants. Term infants double their birth weight by age 4 months and triple their birth weight by age 12 months.

Term infants grow approximately 25 cm in length during the first year, 12.5 cm in the second year, and then slow down to about 5 to 6 cm per year between age 4 and the onset of puberty, at which time growth can increase up to 12 cm per year. Average head circumference is 35 cm at birth and increases rapidly to 47 cm by age 1 year. The rate of growth then slows, reaching an average of 55 cm by age 6 years.

Adjusted growth curves for different populations exist, including those for premature infants, Down syndrome, Turner syndrome, meningomyelocele, intrauterine growth retardation, low birth weight, and very low birth weight. While plotting growth charts for premature patients, a "corrected age" is used when using a standard growth curve. This corrected age is calculated by subtracting the number of weeks of prematurity from the postnatal age (gestational age). This corrected age should be continued with subsequent measurements because it may take an average of 18 months to catch up on head circumference, 24 months for weight, and 40 months for height.

Accurate measurements are essential to the interpretation of growth charts. Scales need to be calibrated regularly, and it helps to use the same machines, if possible, for consecutive measurements. Similarly, lengths should be measured carefully, and head circumference should be measured using standardized techniques.

As long as the patient is growing along a curve (albeit at a lower percentile), FTT should not be diagnosed. Growth variation in normal infants can confound the diagnosis of FTT. About 25% of children will shift their weight or height downward by more than 25 percentile points in the first 2 years of life. These children are falling to their genetic potential or demonstrating constitutional growth delay. After shifting downward, these infants grow at a normal rate along their new percentile and do not have FTT.

In the United States, reports from 1980 to 1989 indicate that FTT accounted for 1% to 5% of tertiary hospital admissions for infants younger than 1 year. This probably represents an underestimation, however, because most children with FTT are not admitted to the hospital. An estimated 10% of children in primary care settings show signs of FTT. In underdeveloped countries, FTT is more common, with malnutrition manifesting as FTT.

Ultimate physical growth may be decreased in children with FTT. Cognitive development is affected in children younger than 5 years who have FTT. Even with improvement of nutritional status, these deficits might not be completely reversed. Traditionally, it had been thought that nonorganic causes of FTT, such as neglect, resulted in more cognitive deficits than organic causes, such as gastrointestinal absorptive problems. In developing countries, malnutrition is a significant cause of mortality, whether directly or secondary to complications such as infection.

FTT can occur in all socioeconomic strata, although it is more frequent in families living in poverty. Studies indicate an increased incidence in children receiving Medicaid, children living in rural areas, and homeless children. Nonorganic FTT is more commonly reported in females than in males.

Causes of Failure to Thrive

Traditionally, FTT has been divided into **organic** and **nonorganic** causes. This distinction is not used as often because most children with FTT have mixed causes. A child with a medical disorder may develop feeding problems, which can cause family stress, which then further compounds the feeding problem. Nonorganic causes may also result from environmental factors, psychological factors, an abnormal interaction between the caregiver and child, or maternal rejection or neglect of the child. A malnourished mother or mother with an eating disorder may also result in a child having FTT. Likewise, family dysfunction, a difficult child, or poor parental feeding skills may lead to FTT.

More recently, the classification of FTT has been based on pathophysiology: inadequate caloric intake, inadequate absorption, excess metabolic demand, or defective utilization.

Inadequate Caloric Intake

Behavioral problems affecting eating

Central nervous system (CNS) damage

Congenital anomalies

- Cleft palate
- Congenital heart disease
- Esophageal atresia

- Macroglossia
- Pyloric stenosis

Disturbed parent-child relationship

Incorrect preparation of formula (too dilute/concentrated)

Mechanical feeding difficulties

Neglect

Oromotor dysfunction

Poverty and food shortages

Severe reflux

Unsuitable feeding habits (excessive juices)

Inadequate Absorption

Biliary atresia or liver disease

Celiac disease

Chronic diarrhea

Cow's milk protein allergy

Cystic fibrosis

Food allergy

Inflammatory bowel disease

Lactose intolerance

Necrotizing enterocolitis or short-gut syndrome

Vitamin or mineral deficiencies (scurvy)

Increased Metabolism

Chronic infection

- Human immunodeficiency virus (HIV)
- Other immunodeficiencies

Hyperthyroidism

Hypoxemia

- Chronic lung disease
- Congenital heart defects

Malignancy

Renal disease

Defective Utilization

Congenital infections

Diabetes mellitus

Genetic abnormalities (trisomies 21, 18, 13)

Metabolic disorders

- Amino acid disorders
- Lead poisoning
- Storage diseases

Peripartum drugs (alcohol, cocaine, tobacco)

Other Causes

Gastroesophageal reflux

Growth hormone deficiency

Hypopituitarism

Hypothyroidism

Prematurity

Key Historical Features

✓ Lethargy, fatigue, or activity level below an age-appropriate level

✓ Parental concern over poor feeding or weight gain

✓ Abnormal voiding patterns, especially diarrhea

✓ Prenatal history
  - Maternal smoking or passive smoke exposure
  - Maternal drug use
  - Maternal alcohol consumption
  - Medication use during pregnancy
  - Illness or infection (meningitis, preeclampsia) during pregnancy
  - Intrauterine growth retardation

✓ Birth history
  - Complications
  - Prematurity
  - Small for gestational age

✓ Feeding history
  - Frequency and duration of breastfeeding or formula feeding
  - How formula is prepared
  - Appropriate advancement of diet
  - Types and amounts of solid food
  - Context of parental-child dynamics during feedings
  - Food aversions
  - Food coercion

- • Milk intake
- • Juice intake
- • Number of wet diapers and stools per day
- • Coughing, choking, or breathing problems associated with feeding
- • Significant vomiting after feedings
- • Abdominal pain or distress following feedings

✓ Past/current medical history, especially
- • Developmental milestones
- • Time of onset of puberty
- • Chronic diarrhea
- • Anemia
- • Asthma
- • Congenital heart disease

✓ Family history
- • Postpartum depression
- • Short stature or FTT
- • Cystic fibrosis or metabolic disorders
- • Data on parents' growth history

✓ Social history
- • Parental inexperience or inattention
- • Care providers
- • Siblings
- • Living conditions
- • Family financial situation
- • Stressors
- • Evidence of neglect

Lastly, the child's developmental status should be ascertained at the time of the visit because children with FTT have a higher incidence of delays than the general population. Physicians should still be concerned about a child without developmental delays who is failing to thrive. FTT is primarily a growth disorder, not a developmental problem.

Key Physical Findings

✓ Vital signs

✓ Height, weight, and head circumference plotted on a growth curve and compared with previous measurements. A corrected age should be used for preterm infants. Charts for special populations should be used when appropriate.

✓ General examination for dysmorphic features suggestive of a genetic disorder impeding growth or any evidence of underlying disease impairing growth

✓ The general assessment should also evaluate for signs of wasting, as well as an assessment of the severity and possible effects of malnutrition

✓ Head and neck examination for craniofacial abnormalities such as severe micrognathia, cleft lip, or cleft palate. The quality of tears and dryness of mucous membranes should be noted. The fontanelles should be evaluated to determine whether they are sunken

✓ Cardiopulmonary examination for any evidence of cardiac or pulmonary disease

✓ Abdominal examination for hepatomegaly or mass

✓ Extremity examination for edema

✓ Skin examination for rashes, skin turgor, or skin changes

✓ Musculoskeletal and skin examination for any evidence of physical abuse

✓ Genitourinary examination if sexual abuse is suspected

✓ Neurologic examination for any mental status changes

✓ Interaction between parent and child

Suggested Work-Up

The laboratory assessment has limited value in determining the etiology of FTT. Occasionally, laboratory test results are unexpectedly abnormal, as in the case of chronic urinary tract infections (UTIs), chronic acidosis, renal failure, and blood dyscrasias. Only about 1% of the tests yield abnormal results leading to the cause of FTT.

Some studies advocate the following screening labs:

Complete blood cell count (CBC)	To evaluate for anemia, infection, or malnutrition (decreased total lymphocyte count)
Electrolytes, blood urea nitrogen, (BUN), and creatinine	To evaluate for renal disease
Serum bicarbonate	To evaluate for chronic acidosis
Fasting glucose	To evaluate for diabetes
Liver function tests, including total protein and albumin	To evaluate for liver disease and malnutrition

Serum prealbumin	To evaluate nutritional status
Iron studies (ferritin, iron, total iron binding capacity [TIBC])	To evaluate for iron deficiency
Urinalysis and urine culture	To evaluate for UTI

Additional Work-Up

HIV test	If HIV infection or acquired immune deficiency syndrome (AIDS) is suspected
Sweat chloride test	If cystic fibrosis is suspected
Thyroid stimulating hormone (TSH)	If hyper- or hypothyroidism is suspected
Lead level	If lead poisoning is suspected
Stool studies for ova and parasites	If intestinal infection is suspected
Fecal fat analysis	If malabsorption is suspected
Serum immunoglobulins	If an immune deficiency is suspected
Purified protein derivative (PPD)	If tuberculosis is suspected
Selected radiologic studies	If abuse or infection is suspected
Serum insulin-like growth factor	If growth hormone deficiency is suspected
Tissue transglutaminase antibody, gliadin antibody, and endomesial antibody	If celiac disease is suspected
Radiologic evaluation for bone age	To help distinguish genetic short stature from constitutional delay of growth
Small intestine biopsy	To confirm a diagnosis of celiac disease

Observing the interaction between the caregiver and child may also give a clue to the cause of FTT. Parents may be asked to feed the child when he or she is hungry while the medical team observes. The caregiver's ability to recognize the child's cues, the child's responsiveness, parental warmth, and appropriate behavior toward the child should all be noted. It is also important to notice the child's temperament and responses toward the parent.

Most children with FTT can be treated as outpatients. Home visits or close clinical follow-up can help determine the underlying cause of FTT and ensure proper treatment. Hospitalization is sometimes necessary for diagnostic or therapeutic reasons (dehydration, infection, anemia, electrolyte imbalances, and unstable home environment). It also allows for direct observation of the parent-child relationship. Hospitalization is also appropriate for children who do not respond to initial management and consists of a multidisciplinary approach including physicians, nurses, dieticians, social workers, and psychologists.

References

1. Adamkin DH. Feeding problems in the late preterm infant. *Clin Perinatol* 2006;33(4):831–837.
2. Allen RE. Nutrition in toddlers. *Am Fam Physician* 2006;74(9):1527–1532.
3. Block RW, Kres NF, and the Committee on Child Abuse and Neglect and the Committee on Nutrition. Failure to thrive as a manifestation of child neglect. *Pediatrics* 2005;116:1234–1237.
4. Corbett SS, Drewett RF, Wright CM. Does a fall down a centile chart matter? The growth and development sequelae of mild failure to thrive. *Acta Paediatr* 1996;85:1278–1283.
5. Frank D, Zeisel S. Failure to thrive. *Pediatr Clin North Am* 1988;35:1187–1205.
6. Gahagan S, Holmes R. A stepwise approach to evaluation of undernutrition and failure to thrive. *Pediatr Clin North Am* 1998;45:169–187.
7. Gubitosi-Klug RA. Idiopathic short stature. *Endocrinol Metab Clin North Am* 2005;34(3):565–580.
8. Krugman SD, Dubowitz H. Failure to thrive. *Am Fam Physician* 2003;68:879–884.
9. Maggioni A, Lifshitz F. Nutritional management of failure to thrive. *Pediatr Clin North Am* 1995;42:791–810.
10. Marsden D. Newborn screening for metabolic disorders. *J Pediatr* 2006;148:577–584.
11. Rudolph CD. Feeding disorders in infants and children. *Pediatr Clin North Am* 2002;49(1):97–112.
12. Schechter M. Weight loss/failure to thrive. *Pediatr Rev* 2000;21:238–239.
13. Shah MD. Failure to thrive in children. *J Clin Gastroenterol* 2002;35:371–374.
14. Sills RH. Failure to thrive: the role of clinical and laboratory evaluation. *Am J Dis Child* 1978;132:967–969.
15. Smith MM, Lifshitz F. Excess fruit juice consumption as a contributing factor in nonorganic failure to thrive. *Pediatrics* 1994;93:438–443.

Jonathan M. Wong

Febrile seizures are common, occurring in 2% to 5% of children in North America at least once in their lifetime. Most of these (65% to 90%) are "simple" febrile seizures (see below). The typical age for febrile seizures ranges from 6 months to 5 years, with a peak occurrence at 18 to 24 months of age.

In 1993, the International League Against Epilepsy defined a febrile seizure as "an epileptic seizure occurring in childhood associated with fever, but without evidence of intracranial infection or defined cause. Seizures with fever in children who have experienced a previous non-febrile seizure are excluded." The evaluation of a febrile seizure is based upon the nature of the seizure and the underlying illness triggering the fever.

Febrile seizures can be classified as either **simple** or **complex**. *Simple febrile seizures* last less than 15 minutes, occur once in a 24-hour period, are generalized, or occur in children with no previous neurologic problems. *Complex febrile seizures* last 15 minutes or longer, occur more than once in a 24-hour period, are focal, or occur in a patient with known neurologic problems such as cerebral palsy.

Although they are frightening, febrile seizures for the most part are benign events. The recurrence rate is approximately 33%. The rate of developing epilepsy is only slightly increased compared with the general population, especially if there are no major risk factors for developing epilepsy. Attention should be paid to relieving parental anxiety and reassuring them of the benign nature of febrile seizures. Parents should be taught what to do in case of a recurrent seizure regarding supportive care and preserving the airway.

Continuous therapy after a febrile seizure is not effective in reducing the development of afebrile seizures. Furthermore, current guidelines do not recommend the use of continuous or intermittent therapy with neuroleptics or benzodiazepines after a simple febrile seizure.

Risk factors for febrile seizure include daycare attendance, developmental delay, a first- or second-degree relative with history of febrile seizure, a history of a neonatal nursery stay of more than 30 days, and male sex (1.4:1 risk). In children with a febrile illness, the height of the fever, the rate of development of the fever, and a family history of febrile seizure affect the likelihood of having a febrile seizure; 10% of siblings and 10% of offspring of a person with febrile seizures in childhood will have a febrile seizure.

Risk factors for recurrent febrile seizure include age younger than 18 months of age at first febrile seizure, short duration of the fever before onset of fever, family history of epilepsy, family history of febrile seizures, and the height of the fever.

Risk factors for the development of afebrile seizures after an episode of febrile seizure include a complex febrile seizure, duration of fever less than 1 hour before onset of febrile seizure, family history of epilepsy, and neurodevelopmental abnormalities such as cerebral palsy or hydrocephalus.

Key Historical Features

✓ Details of the seizure itself (length of time, focal versus generalized)

✓ Length of time between development of fever and onset of the seizure

✓ Temperature measurement if it was performed

✓ Recent illness

✓ Recent antibiotic therapy

✓ Recent immunizations

✓ Medical history

- Birth history
- Neurologic problems
- Developmental delay
- Diabetes
- Neonatal nursery stay

✓ Medications

✓ Family history, especially a first- or second-degree relative with a history of febrile seizure

✓ Social history, especially daycare attendance

Key Physical Findings

✓ Vital signs

✓ General assessment of well-being

✓ Thorough examination for source of the fever

✓ Head and neck examination for otitis, pharyngitis

✓ Abdominal examination for gastroenteritis or peritonitis

✓ Skin examination for viral exanthem or other rashes

✓ Detailed neurologic examination, including funduscopic examination for papilledema

✓ Evaluation for meningeal signs

✓ Evaluation for signs of trauma or intoxication

Suggested Work-Up

A work-up is generally unnecessary unless an evaluation for a source of fever is indicated. The American Academy of Pediatrics recommends that the following determinations not be performed routinely in the evaluation of a first simple febrile seizure: serum electrolytes, calcium, phosphorus, magnesium, complete blood cell count (CBC), or blood glucose. If vomiting and diarrhea accompany a febrile seizure, an assessment of electrolyte concentrations and serum glucose levels may be required. However, the following laboratory tests may be indicated in certain circumstances:

Lumbar puncture with cerebrospinal fluid analysis	Should be considered in children younger than 18 months because meningeal signs are less reliable in this group. Lumbar puncture should also be considered if the patient's mental status is not improving. Lumbar puncture is recommended in infants younger than 12 months after the first seizure with fever.
CBC with differential	May be indicated in the evaluation of the underlying infection
Serum electrolytes	To evaluate for electrolyte derangement, especially if the patient has diarrhea or vomiting
Glucose	If hypoglycemia or hyperglycemia is suspected
Calcium and magnesium	If calcium or magnesium derangement is suspected
Toxicology screen	To evaluate for drug ingestion if indicated by history or if alcohol intoxication is suspected
Neuroimaging (magnetic resonance imaging [MRI] is the preferred modality)	The American Academy of Pediatrics recommends that neuroimaging not be performed in the routine evaluation of the child with a first simple febrile seizure. However, neuroimaging is indicated in a child with a febrile seizure and evidence of increased intracranial pressure or a history or physical examination suggestive of trauma. Also indicated in cases of possible structural defects (e.g., in cases of microencephaly or spasticity).

Electroencephalography has not been found to be helpful in predicting the likelihood of developing epilepsy later in life.

Additional Work-Up

Several studies have examined children with febrile seizure for the incidence of bacterial infection, including unsuspected meningitis. None of these studies reported any cases of meningitis (less than 3% had *Streptococcus pneumoniae* bacteremia, and 3% to 6% had urinary tract infection [UTI]). The absence of any remarkable findings on history or physical examination makes meningitis quite unlikely to be the cause of fever and subsequent seizure.

References

1. Baumann RJ. Technical report: treatment of the child with simple febrile seizures. *Pediatrics* 1999;103:86.
2. Committee on Quality Improvement, Subcommittee on Febrile Seizures. Practice parameter: long-term treatment of the child with simple febrile seizures. *Pediatrics* 1999;103:1307–1309.
3. Duffner PK, Baumann RJ. A synopsis of the American Academy of Pediatrics' practice parameters on the evaluation and treatment of children with febrile seizures. *Pediatr Rev* 1999;20:285–287.
4. Millar JS. Evaluation and treatment of the child with febrile seizure. *Am Fam Physician* 2006;73:1761–1764.

Kevin Haggerty and Theodore X. O'Connell

Petersdorf and Beeson[10] defined fever of unknown origin (FUO) as fever persisting for longer than 3 weeks, a documented temperature of greater than 101° F (38.3° C) on several occasions, and an uncertain diagnosis after intensive study for at least 1 week. Subsequently, in 1968, Dechovitz and Moffet[2] defined FUO in children as fever lasting longer than 2 weeks for which no diagnosis could be made. With the advent of more advanced diagnostic modalities, a more contemporary definition in children is a minimum of 14 days of daily documented temperature of 38.3° C or greater without apparent cause, after performance of repeated physical examinations and screening laboratory tests.

The list of possible causes of FUO is extensive and is outlined below. Although the incidence of the causes of FUO in children may change, most investigators have found that infections predominate. New infectious disease etiologies continue to be added to the list of causes of FUO in children: Epstein-Barr virus (EBV), Lyme disease, hepatitis viruses, and human immunodeficiency virus (HIV). Reported cases demonstrate an increase in cases of osteomyelitis of the axial skeleton and infections resulting from different presentations of *Bartonella henselae* infections.

The approach to a patient with unexplained fever begins with a detailed history and physical examination. The history should review general complaints, not discounting seemingly benign symptoms. Additionally, careful attention must be given to an inventory of recent travel history, living environment, diet, pet and animal exposure, and recent medications. Organ involvement may not always be apparent by history or physical examination when a child first presents with prolonged fever. Physical findings may take weeks to develop, and repeated questioning and physical examinations are critical in the management of any child with prolonged fever.

No algorithms for the evaluation of FUO have been established because the differential diagnosis is so extensive. We have listed tests that can be considered in the evaluation of FUO. The tests should be used based on findings from the history and physical examination. As time passes and the fever persists, the evaluation should become more extensive because common causes of fever become less likely. The child with fever of more than 2 weeks' duration often needs to be admitted to the hospital after the initial outpatient evaluation. The pattern of fever can be assessed, the work-up can be expedited, and the possibility of factitious fever can be eliminated.

Medications Associated with Fever of Unknown Origin

Medications commonly cause febrile episodes in children. Drug fever usually develops 7 to 10 days after the initiation of therapy and may be the sole or most prominent reaction to a medication. Theoretically, any new medication may cause drug fever; the following are the most commonly reported medications:

- Carbamazepine
- Cephalosporins
- Cimetidine
- Hydralizine
- Penicillins
- Phenobarbitol
- Quinidine
- Sulfonamides

Causes of FUO

Infectious Causes

- Bacterial infections
  - Brucellosis
  - Cat-scratch disease (*Bartonella henselae*)
  - Diskitis
  - Dysentery (*Yersinia enterocolitica*, *Salmonella* spp., *Campylobacter jejuni*)
  - Intraspinal abscess
  - Leptospirosis
  - Lyme disease
  - Mastoiditis
  - Osteomyelitis
  - Otitis media
  - Pelvic abscess
  - Peritonsillar abscess
  - *Pneumocystis carinii* pneumonia
  - Pneumonia
  - Pyelonephritis
  - Pyogenic hepatic abscess
  - Q fever (*Coxiella burnetii*)
  - Retroperitoneal abscess
  - Rocky mountain spotted fever
  - *Salmonella* (disseminated infection or focal osteomyelitis)
  - Septic bursitis
  - Sinusitis

- Subacute bacterial endocarditis
- Syphilis
- Tonsillitis
- Tracheobronchitis
- Tuberculosis
- Tularemia
- Typhoid fever
- Urinary tract infection (UTI)
- Viral infections
  - Cytomegalovirus (CMV)
  - EBV (most commonly isolated virus)
  - Enterovirus
  - Hepatitis A, B, C
  - HIV
  - Influenza A and B
- Other infectious agents
  - Aspergillosis
  - Blastomycosis
  - *Coccidioides immitis*
  - Cryptococcal infections
  - Ehrlichiosis
  - *Entamoeba histolytica*
  - Histoplasmosis
  - Malaria
  - Toxoplasmosis

Immunodeficiency Diseases

Primary immunodeficiency diseases usually present with repeated infections; however, prolonged fever can be the presenting manifestation before a definite infection has been identified.

- Common variable immunodeficiency
- Leukocyte adhesion deficiency
- Terminal complement component deficiency
- Wiskott-Aldrich syndrome
- X-linked agammaglobulinemia

Neoplastic Causes

- Acute lymphocytic leukemia
- Hodgkin lymphoma
- Neuroblastoma

Rheumatologic Causes

- Behcet's syndrome
- Idiopathic thrombocytopenic purpura
- Infantile-onset multisystem inflammatory disease
- Juvenile dermatomyositis
- Juvenile rheumatoid arthritis
- Mixed connective tissue disease
- Polymyositis
- Prelupus syndromes
- Scleroderma
- Systemic lupus erythematosus
- Systemic sclerosis
- Vasculitis

Miscellaneous Causes

- Central nervous system (CNS) dysfunction
- Diabetes insipidus
- Ectodermal dysplasia
- Factitious fever
- Familial dysautonomia (Riely-Day syndrome)
- Hemophagocytic syndrome
- Infantile cortical hyperostosis (Caffey disease)
- Inflammatory bowel disease
- Kawasaki disease
- Medications
- Mucha-Habermann disease
- Munchausen syndrome by proxy
- Periodic fever syndromes
  - Blau syndrome
  - Familial cold autoinflammatory syndrome
  - Familial cold urticaria syndrome
  - Familial Mediterranean fever
  - Hyperimmunoglobulin D and periodic fever syndrome

- o Muckle-Wells syndrome
- o Neonatal-onset multisystem inflammatory disease
- o PAPA syndrome (pyogenic sterile arthritis, *Pyoderma gangrenosum,* and acne syndrome)
- o Tumor necrosis factor receptor–associated periodic syndrome
- Rhabdomyolysis
- Thyrotoxicosis

Key Historical Features

✓ Onset and pattern of fever

✓ Severity and duration of fever

✓ Review of systems and complaints

- Abdominal pain
- Adenopathy
- Anorexia
- Bowel symptoms or change in bowel frequency
- Chills
- Diarrhea
- Dizziness
- Focal areas of pain
- Genitourinary symptoms
- Headache
- Irritability
- Joint pain
- Joint stiffness
- Joint swelling
- Listlessness
- Myalgias
- Nausea
- Night sweats
- Oral ulcers
- Pallor
- Pharyngitis
- Rash
- Sleep disturbances or changes in sleep patterns
- Weight loss

- • Visual change
- • Vomiting
- • Weakness
✓ Medical history
✓ Surgical history
✓ Medications
✓ Social history
  - • Place of birth
  - • Foreign Travel
  - • Play and living environment (rural areas, camping trips)
  - • Pet and animal exposure
  - • Drug use
  - • Sexual history, including possible sexual abuse
  - • Family structure and caretaker relationships
✓ Family medical history
  - • Leukemia
  - • Paroxysmal febrile syndromes

Key Physical Findings

✓ Vital signs

✓ Nutritional status

✓ Growth curve plots of height and weight

✓ General assessment of overall health

✓ Ocular and funduscopic examination: Pupillary response to light can be impaired in CNS dysfunction; vasculitic lesions may be seen on fundoscopic exam. Disseminated tuberculosis (TB) or toxoplasmosis can produce funduscopic abnormalities. Conjunctivitis is present in a number of illnesses: bulbar conjunctivitis may be seen in infectious mononucleosis, lupus erythematosus may present with palpebral conjunctivitis, and Kawasaki disease can have a predominantly bulbar conjunctivitis.

✓ Oropharyngeal examination: Pharyngeal hyperemia without exudates may be associated with EBV, CMV, toxoplasmosis, tularemia, or leptospirosis infections. Loss of teeth and gingival hypertrophy can be a sign of leukemia or Langerhans histocytosis. The presence of aphthous stomatitis may indicate lupus, mixed connective tissue disease, or vasculitis.

✓ Neck examination for cervical lymphadenopathy

✓ Cardiovascular examination for friction rubs or prominent or new murmurs

✓ Pulmonary examination for rales or consolidation

✓ Abdominal examination for masses, hepatomegaly, splenomegaly, or focal tenderness

✓ Genitourinary examination

✓ Pelvic examination in adolescent females for cervical discharge, cervical motion tenderness, or adnexal tenderness

✓ Musculoskeletal examination for gait, assessment of strength, point tenderness over the bones, joint tenderness, joint effusion, or limited range of motion in the joints. Each joint should be evaluated for swelling, warmth, redness, and range of motion. Long bones must be palpated carefully for bony tenderness. The spine should be palpated and assessed for range of motion.

✓ Skin examination for rash, petechiae, jaundice (hepatitis, malaria), seborrhea (histoplasmosis), erythrema nodosum (Coccidioides immitis), changes in dermal thickness, tightening or contractures, pigmentation changes, nail changes, or alopecia.

✓ Rectal examination for bloody stool or lesions

✓ Neurologic examination for focal deficits, changes in mental status, ataxia, or seizure activity

Initial Work-Up

During the first week, common causes of fever should be excluded through screening tests and cultures. After the first week of fever, the work-up typically becomes more extensive and no longer is focused on the common infections. The history and physical examination should help guide the tests that are ordered. Tests from each of the following lists may be included or excluded at any time during the evaluation of FUO, as suggested by the clinical findings.

Complete blood cell count (CBC) with differential and platelet count	To evaluate for leukocytosis (infection or rheumatologic disease), leukemia, or thrombocytopenia
Erythrocyte sedimentation rate (ESR)	To evaluate for inflammatory processes
Electrolytes	To evaluate for metabolic derangements such as acidosis

Urinalysis and urine culture	To evaluate for cystitis, pyelonephritis, or inflammatory nephritis
Liver function tests	To screen for hepatitis
Hepatitis screening tests	To evaluate for viral hepatitis
Blood cultures	To evaluate for bacteremia and subacute bacterial endocarditis
Streptococcal enzyme titers	To evaluate for exposure to *Streptococcus* spp.
Lyme titers	To evaluate for Lyme disease, especially in endemic areas or if there is a history of travel to an endemic area
Antinuclear antibody	To evaluate for rheumatologic processes
Purified protein derivative (PPD)	To evaluate for exposure to TB
Chest radiograph	To evaluate for cardiac and pulmonary disease

Additional Work-Up

C-reactive protein	If an inflammatory process is suspected, as an alternative test to the ESR
Thyroid-stimulating hormone (TSH) and thyroxine (T_4)	If thyrotoxicosis is suspected
Stool cultures	If enteritis or typhoid fever is suggested by history
Total protein and albumin	To evaluate nutritional status and hepatic synthetic function
IgG, IgM, and IgA	If immunodeficiency is suspected
IgD	To evaluate for hyperimmunoglobulin D syndrome

Rheumatoid factor	If juvenile rheumatoid arthritis is suspected
HIV test	If HIV infection is suspected
EBV titers	If EBV infection is suspected
CMV screening	If CMV infection is suspected
Urine vanillylmandelic acid (VMA) and metanephrines	If pheochromocytoma is suspected
Stool guaiac testing	If enteritis is suspected
Sweat chloride test	If cystic fibrosis is suspected
Venereal Disease Research Laboratory (VDRL)	To evaluate for syphilis
Lumbar puncture with Gram stain, cell counts, cultures, and viral studies	If CNS infection or inflammation is suspected.
Bartonella titer	If cat-scratch disease is suspected
Toxoplasmosis titer	If toxoplasmosis is suspected
Rickettsia titer	If Rickettsial infection is suspected
Francisella titer	If tularemia is suspected
Coxiella titer	If Q fever is suspected
Candida skin test	To test cellular immunity if primary immunodeficiency is suspected
Synovial fluid analysis evaluation	If a single joint is swollen
Synovial biopsy	If a single joint is swollen and the tuberculin test is positive to evaluate for tuberculous arthritis
Lymph node biopsy	If persistent lymphadenopathy is present and a diagnosis has not been determined

Bone marrow biopsy	If an oncologic process or bone marrow infiltrative process is suspected
Bone biopsy	If a bony lesion is found on imaging study
B-lymphocyte quantification and antibody titers against protein antigens such as tetanus	To test humoral immunity if primary immunodeficiency is suspected
Total hemolytic complement levels	If congenital complement deficiency is suspected
Thick and thin smears for malaria	If malaria is suspected

Imaging Studies

Electrocardiogram (ECG) and echocardiogram	If endocarditis, myocarditis, or pleural effusion is suspected
Radiographs of specific bones	If osteomyelitis or tumor is suspected
Sinus x-rays or computed tomography (CT)	If sinusitis is suspected
Bone scan	To evaluate for osteomyelitis or juvenile arthritis
CT scan of the abdomen	To evaluate for intra abdominal abscess or tumor
Abdominal ultrasound	To evaluate for intra abdominal abscess or tumor
Gallium scan	To evaluate for intra abdominal abscess or tumor
CT scan of the chest	If thoracic pathology is suspected
CT scan or magnetic resonance imaging (MRI) of the brain	If CNS tumor or abscess is suspected

Electroencephalography	If encephalitis is suspected
MRI of the spine	To evaluate for tumor, abscess, or diskitis
MRI of the abdomen	To evaluate for abscess
Vesicoureterogram or intravenous pyelogram	If urinary tract pathology is suspected
Barium enema	If colonic pathology is suspected
Colonoscopy with biopsy	If inflammatory bowel disease is suspected

References

1. Baraff LJ. Management of fever without source in infants and children. *Ann Emerg Med* 2000;36:602–614.
2. Dechovitz AB, Moffet HL. Classification of acute febrile illnesses in childhood. *Clin Pediatr* 1968;7:649–653.
3. Finkelstein JC, Christiansen CL, Platt R. Fever in pediatric primary care: occurrence, management, and outcomes. *Pediatrics* 2000;105:260–265.
4. Ishimine P. Fever without source in children 0 to 36 months of age. *Pediatr Clin North Am* 2006;53:167–194.
5. Jacobs RF, Schutze GE. *Bartonella henselae* as a cause of prolonged fever and fever of unknown origin in children. *Clin Infect Dis* 1998;26:80–84.
6. Miller L, Sisson BA, Tucker LB, Schaller JG. Prolonged fevers of unknown origin in children: patterns of presentation and outcome. *J Pediatr* 1996;12:419–421.
7. Miller ML, Szer I, Yogev R, Bernstein B. Fever of unknown origin. *Pediatr Clin North Am* 1995;42:999–1015.
8. Padeh S. Periodic fever syndromes. *Pediatr Clin North Am* 2005;52:577–609.
9. Palazzi DL, McClain KL, Kaplan SL. Hemophagocytic syndrome in children: an important diagnostic consideration in fever of unknown origin. *Clin Infect Dis* 2003;36:306–312.
10. Petersdorf RG, Beeson PB. Fever of unexplained origin: report on 100 cases. *Medicine* (Baltimore) 1961;40:1–30.

19 GYNECOMASTIA

Theodore X. O'Connell

Gynecomastia, the occurrence of mammary tissue in the male, is a common condition. *True gynecomastia,* the presence of glandular breast tissue, should be distinguished from *pseudogynecomastia,* which is simply adipose tissue seen in overweight boys. Gynecomastia is considered the result of an imbalance between estrogens and androgens.

Gynecomastia occurs in three distinct peaks throughout the life cycle. The first is found in the neonatal period, in which palpable breast tissue transiently develops in 60% to 90% of all newborns because of the transplacental passage of estrogens. The effect disappears in a few weeks. The second peak occurs during puberty, when approximately two thirds of boys develop various degrees of subareolar hyperplasia of the breasts. A rise is seen beginning at approximately the age of 10 and peaks between the ages of 13 and 14, followed by a decline during the late teenage years. Tenderness of the breast is common but transitory. Spontaneous regression may occur within a few months, and gynecomastia rarely persists longer than 2 years. The last peak is found in the adult population, with the highest prevalence among 50- to-80-year-olds.

Benign, self-limited, and usually transitory gynecomastia has been reported in prepubertal children during the initiation of therapy with human growth hormone (HGH). Occasionally, breast development may mimic female breast development and fails to regress, as has been reported in familial gynecomastia. Asymmetric gynecomastia is common, and unilateral gynecomastia may actually represent a stage in the development of bilateral disease.

Prepubertal gynecomastia is uncommon, so an exogenous source of estrogens must be sought. Pathologic causes should be considered. However, a specific cause is rarely identified, and in 90% of patients, prepubertal gynecomastia is labeled idiopathic. Accidental or therapeutic exposure to small amounts of exogenous estrogens by inhalation, percutaneous absorption, or ingestion may cause gynecomastia. Gynecomastia has been observed in children with congenital virilizing adrenal hyperplasia, with Leydig cell tumors of the testes, and with feminizing tumors of the adrenal gland. Gynecomastia also occurs in patients with Klinefelter syndrome, certain types of male pseudohermaphroditism, androgen insensitivity syndromes, and 17-ketosteroid reductase defect.

In patients with Klinefelter syndrome, the risk of breast cancer is 16 times higher than in other men. Male breast cancer is rare, and it is even rarer in the adolescent population but warrants mention. Male breast cancer usually presents as a unilateral eccentric mass, hard or firm, that is fixed to the underlying tissues. It may be associated with dimpling of the skin, retraction or crusting of the nipple, nipple discharge, or axillary lymphadenopathy.

Medications Associated with Gynecomastia

Amiodarone

Anabolic steroids

Angiotensin-converting enzyme inhibitors

Calcium-channel blockers

Chemotherapy agents

- Alkylating agents
- Busulfan
- Imatinib
- Nitrosureas
- Vincristine

Cimetidine

Cisplatin

Clomiphene

Diazepam

Diethylstilbestrol

Digoxin

Efavirenz

Estrogens

Ethionamide

Etomidate

Finasteride

Flutamide

Furosemide

Gonadotropins

Growth hormone

Haloperidol

Isoniazid

Ketoconazole

Melatonin

Methadone

Methotrexate

Methyldopa

Metoclopramide

Metronidazole

Omeprazole

Paroxetine

Pencicillamine

Phenothiazines

Phenytoin

Progesterones

Ranitidine

Reserpine

Risperidone

Spironolactone

Sulindac

Theophylline

Tricyclic antidepressants

Warfarin

Causes of Gynecomastia

Physiologic

Involutional

Neonatal

Pubertal

Pathologic

Adrenal disease

Alcohol abuse

Amphetamine use

Chronic renal failure and dialysis

Congenital defects

- 17-ketosteroid reductase defect
- 3β-hydroxysteroid dehydrogenase defect
- Androgen resistance
- Anorchia
- Defects of testosterone synthesis

Hermaphroditism

Heroin use

Human immunodeficiency virus (HIV) infection

Hyperthyroidism

Idiopathic

Increased estrogen production

Klinefelter's syndrome

Lavender oil exposure

Liver disease

Malnutrition

Marijuana use

Medications

Pseudohermaphroditism (especially Reifenstein syndrome)

Soy products

Tea tree oil exposure

Testicular failure

- Castration
- Granulomatous disease
- Neurologic disease
- Testicular tumors
- Thyrotoxicosis
- Trauma
- Viral orchitis

Key Historical Features

✓ Age

✓ Onset

✓ Rate of growth

✓ Pain or tenderness

✓ Medical history

✓ Medications

✓ Alcohol use

✓ Drug use

Key Physical Findings

✓ Differentiate pseudogynecomastia (fatty tissue) from true gynecomastia

- The patient is placed in the supine position. Then the examiner grasps the breast between the thumb and forefinger and gently moves the two digits toward the nipple. If gynecomastia is present, a firm or rubbery, mobile, disklike mound of tissue arising concentrically from beneath the nipple and areolar region will be appreciated. If the enlargement is due to adipose tissue deposition, no such disk of tissue will be apparent.

✓ Examination of the testes

✓ Evidence of systemic disease, such as thyrotoxicosis, liver disease, or adrenal disease

Suggested Work-Up

Neonatal gynecomastia develops in 60% to 90% of all newborns because of the transplacental passage of estrogens; the effect disappears in a few weeks, and no evaluation is necessary.

Painful, tender gynecomastia appearing during mid-to-late puberty requires only a history and physical examination, including careful palpation of the testicles. If the results are normal, reassurance may be provided and periodic follow-up scheduled. In most boys, the condition resolves spontaneously within 1 to 2 years. No further evaluation is necessary.

Prepubertal gynecomastia is rare and should always be considered pathological, prompting a search for an exogenous or endogenous source of estrogen. In 90% of cases, an underlying cause is not identified. The following is a suggested evaluation:

Thyroid-stimulating hormone (TSH)	To evaluate for hyperthyroidism
Luteinizing hormone	See Figure 19-1
Testosterone level	See Figure 19-1
Estradiol level	To evaluate for testicular Leydig-cell tumor or feminizing adrenocortical neoplasm
Human chorionic gonadotropin (hCG) level	To evaluate for testicular germ cell tumor, extragonadal germ cell tumor, or hCG-secreting nontrophoblastic neoplasm
	See Figure 19-1
Serum electrolytes	To evaluate for adrenal disease
Blood urea nitrogen (BUN) and creatinine	To evaluate for renal disease
Liver function tests	To evaluate for liver disease

Additional Work-Up

Prolactin level	If gynecomastia is associated with galactorrhea to evaluate for prolactinoma
HIV test	If HIV infection is suspected or the patient has risk factors for infection

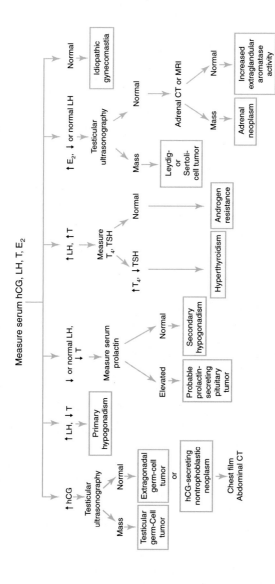

Figure 19-1. Interpretation of serum hormone levels and recommendations for further evaluation of patients with gynecomastia.

Testicular ultrasonongraphy	If testicular examination is abnormal or if estradiol is increased with a decreased or normal luteinizing hormone
Adrenal computed tomography (CT) or magnetic resonance imaging (MRI)	If adrenal neoplasm is suspected

References

1. Braunstein GD. Gynecomastia. *N Engl J Med* 1993;328:490–495.
2. Einav-Bachar R, Phillip M, Aurbach-Klipper Y, Lazar L. Prepubertal gynaecomastia: aetiology, course, and outcome. *Clin Endocrinol (Oxf)* 2004;61:55–60.
3. Henley DV, Lipson N, Korach KS, Bloch CA. Prepubertal gynecomastia linked to lavender and tea tree oils. *N Engl J Med* 2007;356:479–485.
4. Rapaport R. Gynecomastia. In: Behrman RE, Kliegman RM, Jenson HB, eds. *Nelson Textbook of Pediatrics*, 17th ed. Philadelphia: WB Saunders; 2004.
5. Wilson JD. Endocrine disorders of the breast. In: Isselbacher KJ Braunwald E, Wilson JD, eds. *Harrisons's Textbook of Internal Medicine*, 13th ed. New York: McGraw-Hill; 1994:2037–2039.
6. Wise GJ, Roorda AK, Kalter R. Male breast disease. *J Am Coll Surg* 2005;200:255–269.

Timothy J. Horita

Headache is common among children and adolescents: 8% to 12% of 3-year-olds have been reported to have headaches, and the prevalence of headaches has been reported to be as high as 60% to 69% by the age of 7 to 9 years and 75% by 15 years of age. Before puberty, boys are affected more frequently than girls, but after the onset of puberty, headaches occur more frequently in girls.

Despite parental concerns, most cases can be established with an accurate history and physical examination. A detailed history and physical examination are usually all that is needed to make an accurate diagnosis. Children with serious underlying conditions usually have historical features or findings on the neurologic examination that suggest a serious cause. Laboratory tests, imaging studies, and electroencephalogram (EEG) are seldom required to make the diagnosis.

A useful clinical classification system for headache in children is to categorize the headache into one of five temporal patterns: acute, acute recurrent, chronic progressive, chronic nonprogressive, and mixed patterns. The potential causes of each pattern of headache are outlined in the following paragraphs.

Acute headache is a single episode of head pain, often without a history of similar previous events. In children this clinical pattern most often is due to a febrile illness related to an upper respiratory tract infection. Migraine headache is another common cause of acute headache.

Acute recurrent headache occurs when there are recurring episodes of head pain separated by symptom-free intervals. Most acute recurrent headaches in children are either migraine or tension-type headaches. The International Headache Society diagnostic criteria for migraine headache are outlined in Table 20-1. The diagnostic criteria for pediatric migraine without aura are outlined in Table 20-2. The diagnostic criteria for episodic tension-type headache are outlined in Tables 20-3 and 20-4.

Chronic progressive headaches are headaches that gradually increase in frequency and severity over time. This pattern of headache is the most worrisome and, if accompanied by neurologic symptoms or an abnormal neurologic examination, is indicative of increasing intracranial pressure. Potentially worrisome symptoms are outlined in the Key Historical Features section below. The 1991 Childhood Brain Tumor Consortium study published a report of 3291 children diagnosed with brain tumors. Of these children, 62% had headaches before the diagnosis; 98% of the children with headaches had at least one other associated symptom or abnormal sign present. The most frequent symptoms were nausea or vomiting, visual symptoms, difficulty walking, extremity weakness, and changes in personality, academic performance, or speech. The most frequent abnormal neurologic findings were papilledema, abnormal eye movements, ataxia, abnormal tendon reflexes, and defects in the visual examination.

Chronic nonprogressive headache, also called *chronic daily headache,* is defined as 15 or more headaches per month for 4 or more months and the headache usually lasts 4 hours or longer. Adolescents may complain of continuous, unremitting headaches. Neurologic examination is normal. These headaches may result from migraine or tension-type headaches transforming over time to a chronic condition. In children, the period of transformation from first migraine to chronic daily headache is, on average, 2 years, which contrasts with 10 years in adults. Another type of chronic daily headache is persistent daily headache, in which there is often a preceding viral infection or trauma followed by a mysterious onset of daily headache. A fourth and rare form of chronic daily headache is *hemicrania continua,* in which headache occurs for short bursts daily, is responsive to indomethacin, and is always unilateral. Common to all four of these categories of the chronic daily headache pattern is the absence of a positive work-up and the possibility that the condition was exacerbated by medication overuse.

The *mixed headache pattern* implies migraine attacks or analgesic abuse headaches superimposed on a chronic daily pattern.

The primary headache types are very similar to those encountered in older teens and adults. Tension-type headache and migraine are by far the most common causes of episodic headache. They are almost equally prevalent. Migraine, however, can be quite a diagnostic challenge as it can often present atypically. Recognizing the patterns of pediatric migraine is crucial because many of these headaches are "migrainous" without meeting criteria for migraine. There are numerous secondary headache types, but these are much less common. A small subset represents potentially serious causes, but usually several clues or "red flags" are present. The more sinister causes are rarely subtle to the informed clinician; almost all children with a mass lesion have objective findings.

A. At least two attacks fulfilling criteria B-D
B. Aura consisting of at least one of the following, but no motor weakness:
  1. Fully reversible visual symptoms including positive features (i.e., flickering lights, spots, lines) and/or negative features (i.e., scotoma)
  2. Fully reversible sensory symptoms including positive features (i.e., pins and needles) and/or negative features (i.e., numbness)
  3. Fully reversible dysphasic speech disturbance
C. At least two of the following:
  1. Homonymous visual symptoms and/or unilateral sensory symptoms
  2. At least one aura symptom develops gradually over ≥5 min and/or different symptoms occur in succession over = 5 min
  3. Each symptom lasts ≥5 min and ≥60 min

Table 20-1. Continued

D. This criterion determines the subdiagnosis of migraine with typical aura:
   1. Typical aura with migraine headache: headache fulfilling criteria B-D for 1.1 Migraine without aura begins during the aura or follows aura within 60 min, or
   2. Typical aura with nonmigraine headache: headache that does not fulfill criteria B-D for 1.1 Migraine without aura begins during the aura or follows aura within 60 min, or
   3. Typical aura without headache: headache does not occur during the aura nor follow aura within 60 min
E. Not attributed to another disorder

Table 20-1. International Headache Society Diagnostic Criteria for Migraine with Aura

A. 5 attacks fulfilling features B–D
B. Headache attack lasting 1-72 h
C. Headache has at least 2 of the following 4 features:
   1. Either bilateral or unilateral (frontal/temporal) location
   2. Pulsating quality
   3. Moderate to severe intensity
   4. Aggravated by routine physical activities
D. At least 1 of the following accompanies headache:
   1. Nausea and/or vomiting
   2. Photophobia and phonophobia (may be inferred from their behavior)

Table 20-2. 2004 International Headache Society Criteria for Pediatric Migraine without Aura

A. At least 10 episodes occurring on <1 day/mo on average (<12 days/yr) and fulfilling criteria B-D
B. Headache lasting from 30 min to 7 days
C. Headache has at least two of the following characteristics:
   1. Bilateral location
   2. Pressing/tightening (nonpulsating) quality
   3. Mild or moderate intensity
   4. Not aggravated by routine physical activity such as walking or climbing stairs
D. Both of the following:
   1. No nausea or vomiting (anorexia may occur)
   2. No more than one of photophobia or phonophobia
E. Not attributed to another disorder

Table 20-3. 2004 International Headache Society Diagnostic Criteria for Infrequent Episodic Tension-Type Headache

A. At least 10 episodes occurring on ≥1 but <15 days/mo for at least 3 mo (≥12 and <180 days/yr) and fulfilling criteria B-D
B. Headache lasting from 30 min to 7 days
C. Headache has at least two of the following characteristics:
   1. Bilateral location
   2. Pressing/tightening (nonpulsating) quality
   3. Mild or moderate intensity
   4. Not aggravated by routine physical activity such as walking or climbing stairs
D. Both of the following:
   1. No nausea or vomiting (anorexia may occur)
   2. No more than one of photophobia or phonophobia
E. Not attributed to another disorder

Table 20-4. 2004 International Headache Society Diagnostic Criteria for Frequent Episodic Tension Type Headache

Medications and Drugs Associated with Headache

Some of the medications listed below are infrequently used in pediatrics but are included for thoroughness:

Accutane

Acyclovir

Adalimumab

Albendazole

Alpha methyldopa

Amphotericin

Amyl nitrate

Analgesics (over-the-counter and prescribed)

Antibiotics

- Erythromycin and other macrolides
- Metronidazole
- Quinolones
- Sulfa
- Tetracycline

Anticholinergics

Antidepressants

Antihistamines

Antihyperglycemic agents

Antihypertensive agents

Antipsychotic agents

Antiretrovirals

Antiseizure medications

Antispasmodics

Aspartame

Asthma medications

Atovaquone

Bromocriptine

Caffeine (overuse or withdrawal)

Chloroquine

Corticosteroids

Cyclosporine

Decongestants

Depoprovera

Desmopressin

Diabetic medications

- - Antihyperglycemics
  - Insulin

Dipyridamole

Disulfiram

Drugs of abuse
  - Cocaine
  - Inhalants
  - Methamphetamine
  - Nicotine

Epinephrine

Etanercept

Ethanol

Food nitrates/nitrites

Griseofulvin

Herbal and natural remedies
  - Gingko
  - Ginseng
  - Niacin

Histamine blockers

Hydralazine

Hydroxychloroquine

Infliximab

Insulin

Interferon

Isosorbide mono- or dinitrate

Isotretinoin

Linezolid

Lithium

Lopinavir

Monosodium glutamate (MSG)

Muromonab/CD3

Naltrexone

Nifedipine

Nimodipine

Nitroglycerin

Nonsteroidal anti-inflammatory drugs (NSAIDS)

Oral contraceptives

Oxytocin

Phenylpropanolomine

Praziquantel

Progestins

Quinolones

Ritonavir

Serotonin antagonists
- Granisetron
- Ondansetron

Sodium nitroprusside

Stimulants/attention deficit hyperactivity disorder (ADHD) medications

Sulfasalazine

Sympathomimetics

Tetracycline

Vitamin A

Zidovudine

Causes of Headache

Acute Headache (note that causes of acute headache can also cause acute recurrent headache)

Common causes
- Dental infection
- Fever
- Head trauma
- Migraine
- Otitis media
- Pharyngitis
- Upper respiratory tract infection

Allergic disorders

Brain tumor

Caffeine withdrawal

Carbon monoxide exposure

Cerebral abscess

Cervical spine disorders

Constipation

Depression

Encephalitis

Heavy metal toxicity

Hydrocephalus

Hypercapnia

Hypervitaminosis A or B

Hypertension

Hypoglycemia

Hypoxia

Intoxication

Medications

Meningitis

Ocular headache

Porphyria

Postictal state

Postlumbar puncture headache

School phobia

Subarachnoid or intracranial hemorrhage

Substance abuse

- Amphetamine
- Cocaine

Toxins

- Carbon monoxide
- Lead

VP shunt malfunction

Acute Recurrent Headache

Benign occipital epilepsy

Cluster headache

Migraine headache

Neuralgia

Paroxysmal hemicrania

Short-lasting unilateral neuralgiform headache attacks with conjunctival injection and tearing (SUNCT) syndrome

Tension-type headache

Chronic Progressive Headache

Aneurysm

Hydrocephalus

Hypertension

Infection

- Abscess
- Chronic meningitis
- Encephalitis

Malformations

- Chiari malformation
- Dandy Walker

Medications

Neoplasms

Pseudotumor cerebri

Subdural hematoma

Vascular malformation

Chronic Nonprogressive Headache (Chronic Daily Headache)

Hemicrania continua

Persistent daily headache

Transformed migraine (chronic migraine)

Transformed tension-type headache (chronic tension-type headache)

Mixed Headache

Key Historical Features

✓ Worrisome features and red flags include the following:

- Altered level of consciousness in the setting of a headache
- Sudden onset of symptoms
- Fever or other systemic symptoms
- Vertigo
- Focal numbness or weakness
- Visual disturbance
- Seizure
- Headache worsened with exertion, cough, or Valsalva
- Persistent vomiting
- Head trauma
- Headache worse with laying supine
- Unexplained weight loss

✓ Duration of symptoms

✓ Mode of onset

- ✓ Temporal pattern
- ✓ Frequency of the headache
- ✓ Intensity of the pain
- ✓ Location of the pain
- ✓ Quality of the headache
- ✓ Exacerbating and alleviating factors
- ✓ Nausea with or without vomiting
- ✓ Photophobia
- ✓ Phonophobia
- ✓ Smell sensitivity
- ✓ Declining school performance
- ✓ Days of school missed because of headache
- ✓ Behavioral or mood changes
- ✓ Triggers: stress, food, hunger, fatigue, under/over sleeping
- ✓ Any changes from previous headache pattern
- ✓ Response to treatment
- ✓ Medical history, especially:
  - HIV infection or other immunocompromised states
  - Coagulopathy or other hematologic disease
  - Collagen vascular disease
  - Congenital heart disease
  - Endocrine disorders
  - Hypertension
- ✓ Surgical history
  - Recent head and neck surgery
  - Neurosurgical procedures
- ✓ Medications (especially type and frequency of analgesic use)
- ✓ Family history of headaches, especially migraine headache
- ✓ Social history
  - Tobacco use
  - Alcohol use
  - Illicit drug use
  - Toxin exposure

Key Physical Findings

✓ Vital signs, especially for the presence of fever or hypertension

✓ Measurement of head circumference and evaluation of growth parameters

✓ Visual acuity

✓ Funduscopic examination for papilledema

✓ Thorough neurologic examination, including:

  • Mental status

  • Evaluation of speech, affect, and mood

  • Cranial nerve examination, especially pupils and eye movements

  • Facial asymmetry

  • Motor examination for weakness, asymmetry, and pronator drift

  • Coordination

  • Gait

  • Deep tendon reflexes

  • Sensory examination

  • Romberg sign

✓ Head examination for scalp tenderness, sinus tenderness, lymphadenopathy, or tenderness at the temporomandibular joint. Note the patient's dentition for caries or abscess

✓ Neck examination for thyromegaly or nuchal rigidity

✓ Cardiopulmonary examination

✓ Skin examination for café au lait spots

Suggested Work-Up

Most children with acute headaches with a normal physical examination do not require laboratory tests. For the few children who need further evaluation, the work-up should be directed at the underlying suspected etiology. No imaging studies are needed for acute recurrent headaches or for chronic nonprogressive headaches if the history is typical and the neurologic examination is normal.

Additional Work-Up

Complete blood cell count (CBC) and blood culture	If a serious infectious process is suspected
Lumbar puncture	Necessary if meningitis is suspected

Emergent computed tomography (CT) scan followed by lumbar puncture if the CT is normal	If the patient has altered mental status or focal findings on examination
Magnetic resonance imaging (MRI; preferred) or CT scan	For any child suspected of having an intracranial space-occupying lesion or elevated intracranial pressure. Indications for imaging children with headaches are outlined in Table 20-5
Ventriculoperitoneal (VP) shunt tap	May be required for a child with a VP shunt and headache
Electrocardiogram, electrolytes, and urinalysis	For the child with headache and hypertension
Noncontrast head CT followed by lumbar puncture if CT scan is negative. Consider coagulation studies and a platelet count.	If subarachnoid hemorrhage is suspected
Blood glucose	If hypoglycemia is suspected
Toxicology screen	If drug use or toxin exposure is suspected
Carboxyhemoglobin level	If carbon monoxide exposure is suspected
Lead level	If lead toxicity is suspected
Sinus or dental x-rays	If sinusitis or dental infection is suspected, though empiric therapy is a reasonable alternative to imaging
EEG	May be indicated if complex partial seizures are suspected or the headache is associated with an alteration in consciousness or abnormal involuntary movements

Strongly indicated:
1. Chronic progressive headaches
2. Abnormal neurologic examination
3. Worst headache of life: sudden, thunderclap headache
4. Significant head trauma
5. Presence of VP shunt
6. Meningeal signs + focal findings/altered mental status

Consider if:
1. Headache or vomiting on awakening
2. Unvarying location of headache, especially occipital
3. Persistent headache + no family history of migraine
4. Neurocutaneous syndrome
5. Age <3 yr old (limited verbalization skills)

Table 20-5. Indications for Imaging Children with Headaches

References
1. Anttila P. Tension-type headache in childhood and adolescence. *Lancet Neurol* 2006;5(3):268–274.
2. Gladstein J. Headache. *Med Clin North Am* 2006;90(2):275–290.
3. Headache Classification Subcommittee of the International Headache Society. The international classification of headache disorders, 2nd ed. *Cephalalgia* 2004;24:9–160.
4. Lewis DW. Headaches in children and adolescents. *Am Fam Physician* 2002;65(4):625–632.
5. Lewis DW, Rothner AD. Headache in children and adolescents. In: Johnson RT, Griffin JW, McArthur JC, eds. *Current Therapy in Neurologic Disease*, 6th ed. St. Louis, MO: Mosby; 2002.
6. Lewis DW, et al. Practice parameter: evaluation of children and adolescents with recurrent headache. *Neurology* 2002;59:490–498.
7. Lewis D, et al. Practice parameter: pharmacological treatment of migraine headache in children and adolescents. Report of the American Academy of Neurology Quality Standards Subcommittee and the Practice Committee of the Child Neurology Society. *Neurology* 2004;63:2215–2224.
8. Lipton RB. Classification of primary headaches. *Neurology* 2004;63(3):427–435.
9. Mortimer HJ, Kay J, Jaron A. Epidemiology of headache and childhood migraine in an urban general practice using ad hoc, Vahlquist, and HIS criteria. *Dev Med Child Neurol* 1992;34:1095–1101.
10. Qureshi F. Managing headache in the pediatric emergency department. *Clin Ped Emerg Med* 2003;4:159–170.
11. Sackhara T. Pediatric SUNCT syndrome. *Pediatr Neurol* 2005;33(3):206–207.
12. Schobitz E. Pediatric headaches in the emergency department. *Curr Pain Headache Rep* 2006;10(5):391–396.
13. The Childhood Brain Tumor Consortium. The epidemiology of headache among children with brain tumor. Headache in children with brain tumors. *J Neuro-oncol* 1991;10:31–46.
14. The International Classification of Headache Disorders. 2nd ed. *Cephalalgia* 2004;24:1–160.
15. Wilne S, et al. Presentation of childhood CNS tumours: a systematic review and meta-analysis. *Lancet Oncol* 2007;8(8):685–695.
16. Young WB. Drug-induced headache. *Neurol Clin* 2004;22(1):173–184.
17. Zuckerman B, Stevenson J, Bailey V. Stomach aches and headaches in a community sample of preschool children. *Pediatrics* 1987;79:677–682.

Theodore X. O'Connell

As many as 90% of children will have an audible heart murmur at some time, yet the incidence of structural congenital heart disease is estimated to be less than 1% of all live births. A murmur may be heard in 60% of healthy newborn babies. As such, the physician must determine which patients require further evaluation.

Features of concern in infants include feeding intolerance, failure to thrive, respiratory symptoms, or cyanosis. In older children, chest pain (especially with exercise), syncope, exercise intolerance, or a family history of sudden death in young people should raise the physician's level of suspicion. Other features that increase the likelihood of cardiac pathology include malformation syndromes, increased precordial activity, decreased femoral pulses, abnormal second heart sounds, clicks, a loud or harsh murmur, and increased intensity of the murmur when the patient stands.

The clinical diagnosis of a normal or innocent murmur should occur in the setting of an otherwise normal history, physical examination, and appearance. The innocent systolic murmurs are soft (grade 1 or 2) and ejection in quality. Normal murmurs are never solely diastolic. The intensity of an innocent murmur is grade 3 or less and, consequently, is never associated with a palpable thrill. Most murmurs, both innocent and organic, may be accentuated by fever, anemia, or increased cardiac output.

The pathologic systolic murmur occurs early in systole and can be quite loud. Diastolic murmurs are much less common in children, and the presence of a diastolic murmur indicates that structural heart disease is present and warrants referral. Continuous precordial murmurs in infants are also generally pathologic, with the exception of the venous hum. The venous hum should resolve in the supine position or with gentle compression of the jugular vein. Patients with venous hums do not require pediatric cardiology referral.

Holosystolic murmurs occur when a regurgitant atrioventricular valve is present or in association with most ventricular septal defects. *Ejection murmurs* may arise from narrowing of the semilunar valves or outflow tracts. Innocent murmurs are almost exclusively systolic ejection in nature. They are generally soft, never associated with a palpable thrill, and vary considerably with positional changes. *Early systolic murmurs* are associated exclusively with small muscular ventricular septal defects. *Mid-to-late systolic murmurs* are often heard in association with mitral valve prolapse.

Diastolic murmurs may be associated with regurgitation of the aortic or pulmonary valves, stenosis of an atrioventricular valve, or increased flow across an atrioventricular valve. Early diastolic murmurs arise from either aortic or pulmonary valve insufficiency. Mid-diastolic murmurs occur because of either increased flow across a normal tricuspid valve or mitral valve or normal flow across an obstructed or stenotic tricuspid or mitral valve. Late diastolic or crescendo murmurs are caused by stenotic or narrowed atrioventricular valves.

Specific Lesions

Most innocent heart murmurs in healthy term infants are related to *peripheral pulmonary stenosis*, which is reduced in two thirds of cases by 6 weeks of age and in most others by 6 months. The murmur is soft (grade 1 or 2), ejection in quality, and best heard anteriorly at the left upper sternal border with characteristic transmission to the axillae and back bilaterally. No associated signs or symptoms of heart disease are present. The murmur of atrial septal defect may mimic this murmur but is generally heard in later infancy or childhood. Pathologic peripheral pulmonary stenosis is typically more severe, has a louder murmur, and does not regress over time. If peripheral pulmonary stenosis is suspected in the term infant, close follow-up is indicated. If the murmur intensifies or persists after 6 months of age, cardiology referral is indicated.

Isolated *ventricular septal defects* are the most common congenital heart defect identified through the first three decades of life. Infants with ventricular septal defect can present in different ways, and presentation is determined by the size of the defect and the status of the pulmonary vascular resistance. Most commonly the murmur is detected at 2 to 6 weeks of age. The infant with a small ventricular septal defect may have a loud murmur but appears healthy with normal growth and no cardiac symptoms. The precordial activity is normal, and there typically is no palpable systolic thrill. The infant with a moderate-sized ventricular septal defect often has poor weight gain and may have dsypnea and diaphoresis, particularly with feedings. The murmur is loud, is frequently associated with a systolic thrill, is harsh and holosystolic, and obscures the first and second heart sounds. A prominent third heart sound or diastolic flow murmur can be heard at the cardiac apex. The infant with a large ventricular septal defect has significant clinical symptoms such as feeding problems, failure to thrive, and irritability. The murmur is soft, short, and early systolic. There is a marked right ventricular heave with a loud and single second heart sound. A prominent third heart sound and diastolic rumble are common, and hepatomegaly is usually present. Cardiology referral is indicated for children with suspected ventricular septal defect.

Tetralogy of Fallot refers to a spectrum of abnormalities characterized by a large ventricular septal defect and right ventricular outflow tract obstruction. It is the most common form of cyanotic congenital heart disease and is associated with a higher incidence of extracardiac anomalies and malformation syndromes. The clinical presentation depends on the severity of right ventricular outflow tract obstruction. If the degree of right ventricular outflow tract obstruction is severe, the infant can present with severe cyanosis as the patent ductus arteriosus closes. The right ventricular impulse is increased, there may be a systolic thrill, and the second heart sound is typically single. The murmur can be loud, is ejection in quality, and diminishes in intensity and length when the degree of obstruction increases. If tetralogy of Fallot is suspected, pulse oximetry should be performed. A chest radiograph may demonstrate a boot-shaped heart. Prompt cardiology referral is indicated.

In *pulmonary valve stenosis*, the intensity of the murmur depends on the severity of obstruction. The right ventricular impulse is prominent, and there may be a systolic thrill at the left upper sternal border. An ejection sound is characteristic and is recognized by its high-pitched clicking quality, which varies with respiration. The pulmonic component of the second heart sound is delayed and soft. The murmur is often loud, ejection in quality, and best heard at the left upper sternal border. Cardiology referral is indicated.

Isolated *atrial septal defects* are rarely diagnosed in the neonate. Young children with atrial septal defects often have a thin habitus. Precordial palpation reveals a prominent hyperdynamic right ventricular impulse. Wide, fixed splitting of the second heart sound is the auscultatory hallmark. The murmur is usually grade 2 or 3, systolic ejection in quality, and heard best at the left upper sternal border. A mid-diastolic flow rumble is present. Pulse oximetry should be normal. Cardiology referral is indicated.

Aortic stenosis is much more common in males. Most infants with this lesion are otherwise healthy, with appropriate growth and development, unless severe aortic stenosis is present. The left ventricular impulse can be normal in mild obstruction or increased in more moderate obstruction. A systolic thrill is common and may be appreciated in the suprasternal notch and over both carotid arteries. The murmur is maximal in the second right interspace, with radiation to the right and into the neck. The intensity of the murmur is variable. A louder, longer, late-peaking murmur generally is indicative of more significant obstruction. Cardiology referral is indicated, with more urgent referral in the neonate or young infant.

The hallmark clinical feature of *coarctation of the aorta* is absent or weak femoral pulses. The diagnosis can be confirmed when a higher measured blood pressure is observed in the arm compared with the leg. A systolic ejection click may be heard if there is an associated bicuspid aortic valve. The murmur is generally soft, ejection in quality, and audible at the left upper sternal border and over the left back. Urgent cardiology referral is indicated.

The most common innocent murmur in children is the *vibratory Still's murmur*. The murmur is typically audible between ages 2 and 6 years, but it may be present as late as adolescence or as early as infancy. The murmur is low to medium in pitch, confined to early systole, generally grade 2, and maximal at the lower left sternal edge and extending to the apex. The murmur is generally loudest in the supine position and often changes in character, pitch, and intensity with upright positioning. The most characteristic feature of the murmur is its vibratory quality.

Causes of Heart Murmurs

Innocent Murmurs of Childhood

Aortic systolic murmur

Mammary arterial souffle

Peripheral pulmonary arterial stenosis

Pulmonary flow murmur

Supraclavicular systolic murmur

Venous hum

Vibratory Still's murmur

Pathologic Murmurs of Childhood

Aortic stenosis

Atrial septal defect

Coarctation of the aorta

Hypertrophic cardiomyopathy

Mitral valve regurgitation

Patent ductus arteriosus

Pulmonary stenosis

Subaortic stenosis

Tetralogy of Fallot

Tricuspid valve regurgitation

Ventricular septal defect

Key Historical Features

✓ Pregnancy course and maternal history
- Maternal medication use
- Maternal alcohol or drug use
- Maternal diabetes, especially if poorly controlled
- Chronic or acute maternal illness
- Congenital infections

✓ Perinatal course
- Birth weight
- Problems at the time of birth
- Cyanosis or tachypnea
- Early growth and development

- Feeding history, including volume per feeding and length of time per feeding
- Tachypnea or diaphoresis associated with feedings

✓ Developmental milestones

✓ Family history
- First-degree relative with structural heart disease
- Sudden death, especially in young individuals
- Sudden infant death syndrome (SIDS)
- Rheumatic fever
- Any known heritable syndromes

Key Physical Findings

✓ Vital signs, including heart rate, respiratory rate, and blood pressure

✓ Growth parameters plotted on a growth chart

✓ General assessment of overall appearance

✓ Dysmorphic features or extracardiac anomalies

✓ Assessment for cyanosis

✓ Signs of respiratory distress such as tachypnea, retractions, grunting, or nasal flaring

✓ Cardiac examination
- Inspection and palpation for precordial bulge, substernal heave, or palpable precordial thrill
- Auscultation
  - Auscultation should be performed with the patient in the supine, sitting, and standing positions
  - The first heart sound, which reflects closure of the mitral and tricuspid valves, is typically single and is best heard at the left lower sternal border
  - The second heart sound, which reflects closure of the aortic and pulmonary valves, is split, varies with respiration, and is best heard at the left upper sternal border
  - Third and fourth heart sounds can be normal in the child, are typically low in frequency, and are best heard at the cardiac apex
  - Murmurs should be described by their intensity, timing, location, and radiation. Any variability of the murmur with a change in position or a maneuver should be described

- o Dynamic maneuvers, including respiration, Valsalva, exercise, and postural changes, may provide important diagnostic information
  - Assessment of the peripheral pulses for rate, rhythm, and character (especially the femoral pulses). After the brachial pulses have been palpated, the right brachial pulse should be palpated simultaneously with the femoral pulse
  - Assessment of capillary refill time
✓ Abdominal examination for liver character and size
✓ Extremity examination for pallor or clubbing

Suggested Work-Up

The evaluation of a pediatric heart murmur is based on a thorough history and physical examination, described above. Echocardiography or pediatric cardiology consultation should be based on the suspected cause of the murmur.

References
1. Frommelt MA. Differential diagnosis and approach to a heart murmur in term infants. *Pediatr Clin North Am* 2004;51:1023–1032.
2. Harris JP. Evaluation of heart murmurs. *Pediatr Rev* 1995;12:490–493.
3. McConnell ME, Adkins SB, Hannon DW. Heart murmurs in pediatric patients: when do you refer? *Am Fam Physician* 1999;60:558–565.
4. Pelech AN. Evaluation of the pediatric patient with a cardiac murmur. *Pediatr Clin North Am* 1999;46:167–187.

Theodore X. O'Connell

Gross (macroscopic) hematuria is defined as blood that can be seen with the naked eye. In one study, gross hematuria had an estimated incidence of 1.3 per 1000. In contrast to **microscopic hematuria**, systematic evaluation of gross hematuria often yields results, and most patients have a clinically important cause identified. The source of bleeding may originate from the glomerulus and interstitium, the urinary tract, or the renal vasculature.

Cola-colored urine, red blood cell (RBC) casts, and dysmorphic RBCs suggest glomerular bleeding. Edema, hypertension, and proteinuria are also suggestive of glomerulonephritis. Macroscopic hematuria from the bladder and urethra is usually pink or red. An absence of RBCs in the urine with a positive dipstick reaction suggests hemoglobinuria or myoglobinuria.

The approach to gross hematuria begins with a description of the urine and questions directed toward associated symptoms. Recent illnesses, medication use, and family history also may provide important clues to the diagnosis. Discussion of each of the causes of hematuria is beyond the scope of this chapter but can be found in Meyers.[4]

Asymptomatic gross hematuria presents more of a challenge. All patients with asymptomatic gross hematuria should first have radiologic interrogation to rule out renal and bladder tumors. IgA nephropathy commonly presents with recurrent episodes of painless, gross hematuria, with a mean age of presentation of 9 to 10 years in children. Acute postinfectious glomerulonephritis is the most common form of glomerulonephritis in children, and may be asymptomatic. Gross hematuria may occur after high intensity or long duration exercise.

An algorithm for the approach to gross hematuria is provided in Figure 22-1 in addition to selected tests that may be used in the evaluation.

Medications Associated with Hematuria

- Amitriptyline
- Antibiotics
- Anticoagulants
- Anticonvulsants
- Chlorpromazine
- Cyclophosphamide
- Indinavir
- Nonsteroidal anti-inflammatory drugs (NSAIDs)
- Ritonavir
- Toluene

145

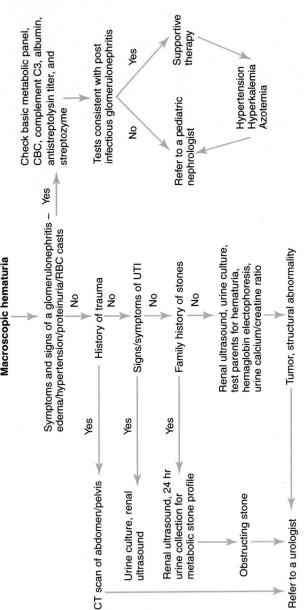

Figure 22-1. Macroscopic hematuria. (From Meyers KEC. Evaluation of hematuria in children. *Urol Clin North Am* 2004;31:559–573, with permission.)

Medications That May Cause Urinary Discoloration
Misinterpreted as Hematuria

- Chloroquine
- Deferoxamine mesylate
- Iron
- Isoniazid
- Melanin
- Methyldopa
- Metronidazole
- Nitrofurantoin
- Pyridium
- Riboflavin
- Rifampin
- Salicylates
- Sulfa

Causes of Hematuria

Bleeding Disorders

- Coagulopathy (congenital or acquired)
- Hemophilia A or B
- Platelet disorder
- Thrombocytopenia
- von Willebrand disease

Glomerular Causes

- Acute poststreptococcal glomerulonephritis
- Alport syndrome
- Bacterial endocarditis
- Goodpasture disease
- Hemolytic uremic syndrome
- Henoch-Schönlein purpura
- Idiopathic hypercalciuria without urolithiasis
- IgA nephropathy
- Membranoproliferative glomerulonephritis
- Mesangial proliferative glomerulonephritis
- Microangiopathic polyarteritis nodosa
- Polycystic kidney disease
- Rapidly progressive glomerulonephritis
- Systemic lupus erythematosus

- Thin basement membrane disease (benign familial hematuria)
- Thrombotic thrombocytopenic purpura
- Wegener granulomatosis

Interstitial Disease

- Acute interstitial nephritis
- Pyelonephritis
- Tubulointerstitial nephritis with uveitis

Neoplastic

- Angiomyolipoma
- Congential mesoblastic tumor
- Renal cell carcinoma
- Rhabdoid tumors
- Uroepithelial tumors
- Wilms' tumor

Urinary Tract

- Bacterial infection
- Cyclophosphamide cystitis
- Cystitis
- Foreign body
- Idiopathic hypercalciuria
- Schistosomiasis
- Severe hydronephrosis
- Trauma
- Tuberculosis
- Urethritis
- Urolithiasis
- Viral (adenovirus)

Vascular

- Ateriovenous thrombosis
- Exercise-related hematuria
- Hemangioma/hamartoma
- Malignant hypertension
- Nutcracker syndrome
- Renal artery or vein thrombosis
- Sickle cell disease and trait
- Trauma

Key Historical Features

✓ Description of the urine

✓ Dysuria

✓ Frequency

✓ Urgency

✓ Fever

✓ Flank pain

✓ Abdominal pain

✓ Trauma

✓ Recent febrile illness

✓ Recent pharyngitis

✓ Recent streptococcal skin infection

✓ Recent trauma, menstruation,
   or strenuous exercise

✓ Past medical history
   • History of heavy or frequent bleeding
   • Exposure to tuberculosis
   • Recent bladder catheterization

✓ Past surgical history

✓ Family history of renal disease, hematuria, hearing loss, coagulopathy,
   hemoglobinopathy, calculi, dialysis, or renal transplantation

✓ Review of systems
   • Shortness of breath
   • Edema
   • Weight gain
   • Chest pain
   • Fatigue
   • Diarrhea
   • Joint pains
   • Rash
   • Cough or hemoptysis
   • Hematochezia
   • Hair loss
   • Mouth ulcers

Key Physical Findings

✓ Vital signs, especially elevated blood pressure or fever

✓ Assessment of growth

✓ General appearance, especially for pallor

✓ Abdominal examination for abdominal or flank masses

✓ Abdominal auscultation for bruits

✓ Back examination for costovertebral angle tenderness

✓ Skin examination for rashes

✓ Extremity examination for musculoskeletal findings such as arthritis

Suggested Work-Up

Urine dipstick	Greater than 2+ proteinuria should raise suspicion for glomerular disease
Urine microscopy	To confirm the presence of RBCs
	Red cell casts may be a clue to glomerulonephritis
	Bacteria and significant pyuria may indicate pyelonephritis or cystitis
Renal ultrasound	Indicated for all children with macroscopic hematuria to evaluate for urologic disease, congenital abnormalities, or renal parenchymal disease
Electrolytes, blood urea nitrogen (BUN), creatinine, complement C3, albumin, anti-streptolysin O titer, and streptozyme	Indicated for symptoms and signs of glomerulonephritis such as edema, complete blood cell count (CBC), hypertension, proteinuria, or RBC casts

Additional Work-Up

CBC, BUN, and creatinine	If glomerulonephritis is suspected
C3, C4, antinuclear antibody, and anti-double-stranded DNA antibody	If systemic lupus erythematosus is suspected

C3, C4, antistreptolysin O, and anti-Dnase B antibody	If poststreptococcal glomerulonephritis is suspected
Antineutrophilic cytoplasmic antibody titer (ANCA)	If Wegener's granulomatosis is suspected
Antiglomerular basement antibody titer	If Goodpasture's syndrome is suspected
Skin biopsy	If Henoch-Schönlein purpura is suspected by the presence of arthralgias, purpura, pedal edema, abdominal pain, and hematochezia
24-hour urine collection for protein or a spot urine protein-creatinine ratio	If proteinuria is present
Urine culture	Indicated in patients who have fever, flank pain, abdominal pain, or bladder pain
24-hour urine collection for calcium or a spot urine calcium-creatinine ratio	If hypercalciuria is suspected. Hypercalciuria is defined as calcium excretion >4 mg/kg per day or a spot urine calcium-creatinine ratio of >0.22. Note that normal values may be greater in children younger than 7 years
Serum IgA	If IgA nephropathy is suspected
Urine eosinophils	If acute interstitial nephritis is suspected
Renal ultrasonography	If urologic disease or congenital abnormalities are suspected
Computed tomography (CT) imaging	May be used to identify kidney stones and provides detailed images of the bladder, pelvis, and retroperitoneum when looking for masses. Indicated promptly if there is a history of abdominal trauma

| Renal biopsy | If the diagnosis remains in doubt after laboratory and radiologic evaluation |
| Urology referral | Required when the clinical evaluation and work-up indicate a tumor, a structural urogenital abnormality, or an obstructing calculus. Referral is also indicated for recurrent nonglomerular macroscopic hematuria of undetermined origin because cystoscopy may be warranted |

References

1. Gordon C, Stapleton FB. Hematuria in adolescents. *Adolesc Med* 2005;16:229–239.
2. Ingelfinger JR, Davis AE, Grupe WE. Frequency and etiology of gross hematuria in a general pediatric setting. *Pediatrics* 1977;59:557–561.
3. Mahan JD, Turman MA, Mentser MI. Evaluation of hematuria, proteinuria, and hypertension in adolescents. *Pediatr Clin North Am* 1997;44:1573–1589.
4. Meyers KEC. Evaluation of hematuria in children. *Urol Clin North Am* 2004;31:559–573.
5. Pan CG. Evaluation of gross hematuria. *Pediatr Clin North Am* 2006;53:401–412.
6. Patel HP, Bissler JJ. Hematuria in children. *Pediatr Clin North Am* 2001;48:1519–1537.

Theodore X. O'Connell

Microscopic hematuria is much more common than gross hematuria in children, with a prevalence of 3% to 4% in a single urine sample and 1% to 2% in two or more urine samples. There is no consensus on the definition of microscopic hematuria, although more than 5 to 10 red blood cells (RBCs) per high-power field is considered significant. It is generally recommended that at least two of three uninalyses show microscopic hematuria over 2 to 3 weeks before further evaluation is performed. No consensus exists on a stepwise evaluation, but this chapter provides an approach to the evaluation of the child with microscopic hematuria.

Hematuria may originate from the glomeruli, renal tubules and interstitium, or urinary tract, which includes the collecting systems, ureters, bladder, and urethra. In children, the source of bleeding is most often from the glomeruli. In most cases, proteinuria, RBC casts, and dysmorphic RBCs in the urine accompany hematuria caused by glomerulonephritis. The most common causes of persistent microscopic hematuria in children include glomerulopathies (e.g., IgA nephropathy, thin basement membrane disease), Alport syndrome, hypercalciuria, and urinary tract infection (UTI).

The presence of hematuria must be confirmed by microscopic examination of the spun sediment of urine because other substances besides blood can give a false-positive dipstick test for blood. The dipstick and microscopic urinalysis should be repeated twice within 2 weeks after the initial specimen. If the hematuria resolves, no further tests are needed. If persistent microscopic hematuria is confirmed, a thorough history (with particular attention to the family history) and physical examination should be performed.

Two diagnostic tests should be performed: a test for proteinuria and a microscopic examination of the urine for RBCs and RBC casts. Proteinuria usually does not exceed 2+ (100 mg/dL) if the only source of protein is from the blood. Patients with 1+ to 2+ proteinuria should be evaluated for orthostatic proteinuria. A patient with more than 2+ proteinuria should be evaluated for glomerulonephritis and nephrotic syndrome. The presence of RBC casts is a highly specific marker for glomerulonephritis. In addition to these tests, many authorities also recommend urine culture, urine calcium-to-creatinine ratio, and renal ultrasound examination for confirmed cases of microscopic hematuria.

Microscopic hematuria that persists falls into one of three categories: asymptomatic isolated microscopic hematuria, asymptomatic microscopic hematuria with proteinuria, and symptomatic isolated microscopic hematuria.

Asymptomatic isolated microscopic hematuria is common in children. Many experts recommend observation of these children if the examination is normal, with further evaluation only if proteinuria, hypertension, or gross hematuria is present. In the child with asymptomatic isolated microscopic hematuria, the early morning urinalysis should be repeated weekly for 2 weeks with no exercise before the collection of the urine sample. If the hematuria persists, urine culture should be obtained and, if positive, the patient should be treated with antibiotics. If the urine culture is negative, the patient should be followed up every 3 months with a history, physical examination, blood pressure measurement, and urinalysis. If the hematuria persists for 1 year, measurement of the urine calcium-creatinine ratio should be obtained, and the parents and siblings should be tested for hematuria. Hemoglobin electrophoresis should be performed if sickle cell trait is a consideration. Figure 23-1 provides an algorithm for the evaluation of a child with asymptomatic microscopic hematuria.

Asymptomatic microscopic hematuria with proteinuria is associated with a higher risk for significant renal disease. In this case, urinary protein excretion should be quantified. If protein excretion is greater than 4 mg/m^2 per hour or the urine protein-to-creatinine ratio is greater than 0.2 mg protein per milligram of creatinine in children older than 2 years or greater than 0.5 mg of protein per milligram of creatinine in younger children, the patient should be referred to a pediatric nephrologist. If urinary protein excretion is less than these values, the patient should be reevaluated in a few weeks. If the hematuria and proteinuria have resolved, no further evaluation is indicated. If there is only asymptomatic microscopic hematuria, the patient may be monitored as for asymptomatic isolated microscopic hematuria. If the hematuria and proteinuria persist, the patient should be referred to a pediatric nephrologist. Additional testing is outlined below. Figure 23-2 provides an algorithm for the evaluation of a child with microscopic hematuria associated with proteinuria, symptoms, or abnormalities in the history or physical examination.

Symptomatic microscopic hematuria may manifest with fever, weight loss, malaise, rash, arthritis, edema, hypertension, dysuria, or oliguria. The presence of these symptoms suggests a systemic process or significant disease affecting the urinary tract. History and physical examination may provide important clues to the diagnosis. The laboratory evaluation includes serum creatinine, blood urea nitrogen (BUN), electrolytes, complete blood count (CBC), C3, C4, and albumin. Additional testing to consider is outlined below. Important causes of symptomatic microscopic hematuria include acute postinfectious glomerulonephritis, hemolytic-uremic syndrome, Henoch-Schönlein purpura, menbranoproliferative glomerulonephritis, IgA nephropathy, and focal segmental glomerulosclerosis.

Medications Associated with Hematuria

- Amitriptyline
- Antibiotics
- Anticoagulants
- Anticonvulsants

- Chlorpromazine
- Cyclophosphamide
- Indinavir
- Nonsteroidal anti-inflammatory drugs (NSAIDs)
- Ritonavir
- Toluene

Causes of Hematuria

Bleeding Disorders

- Coagulopathy (congenital or acquired)
- Hemophilia A or B
- Platelet disorder
- Thrombocytopenia
- von Willebrand disease

Glomerular Causes

- Acute poststreptococcal glomerulonephritis
- Alport syndrome
- Bacterial endocarditis
- Goodpasture's disease
- Hemolytic uremic syndrome
- Henoch-Schönlein purpura
- Idiopathic hypercalciuria without urolithiasis
- IgA nephropathy
- Membranoproliferative glomerulonephritis
- Mesangial proliferative glomerulonephritis
- Microangiopathic polyarteritis nodosa
- Polycystic kidney disease
- Rapidly progressive glomerulonephritis
- Systemic lupus erythematosus
- Thin basement membrane disease (benign familial hematuria)
- Thrombotic thrombocytopenic purpura
- Wegener granulomatosis

Interstitial Disease

- Acute interstitial nephritis
- Pyelonephritis
- Tubulointerstitial nephritis with uveitis

Neoplastic

- Angiomyolipoma
- Congential mesoblastic tumor
- Renal cell carcinoma
- Rhabdoid tumors
- Uroepithelial tumors
- Wilms' tumor

Urinary Tract

- Bacterial
- Cyclophosphamide cystitis
- Cystitis
- Foreign body
- Idiopathic hypercalciuria
- Schistosomiasis
- Severe hydronephrosis
- Trauma
- Tuberculosis
- Urethritis
- Urolithiasis
- Viral (adenovirus)

Vascular

- Arteriovenous thrombosis
- Hemangioma/hamartoma
- Malignant hypertension
- Nutcracker syndrome
- Renal artery or vein thrombosis
- Sickle cell disease and trait
- Exercise-related hematuria
- Trauma

Key Historical Features

✓ Dysuria

✓ Frequency

✓ Urgency

✓ Fever

✓ Flank pain

✓ Abdominal pain

✓ Trauma

✓ Recent febrile illness

✓ Recent pharyngitis

✓ Recent streptococcal skin infection

✓ Recent trauma, menstruation, or strenuous exercise

✓ Medical history
  • History of heavy or frequent bleeding
  • Exposure to tuberculosis
  • Recent bladder catheterization

✓ Surgical history

✓ Family history of renal disease, hematuria, hearing loss, coagulopathy, hemoglobinopathy, calculi, dialysis, or renal transplantation

✓ Review of systems
  • Shortness of breath
  • Edema
  • Weight gain
  • Chest pain
  • Fatigue
  • Diarrhea
  • Joint pains
  • Rash
  • Cough or hemoptysis
  • Hematochezia
  • Hair loss
  • Mouth ulcers

Key Physical Findings

✓ Vital signs, especially blood pressure and temperature

✓ Assessment of growth

✓ General appearance, especially for pallor

✓ Abdominal examination for abdominal or flank masses

✓ Back examination for costovertebral angle tenderness

✓ Skin examination for rashes

✓ Extremity examination for musculoskeletal findings such as arthritis

Suggested General Work-Up of Microscopic Hematuria

Test for proteinuria	To determine whether significant proteinuria is present
Microscopic examination of the urine for RBCs and RBC casts	To confirm the presence of hematuria and evaluate for underlying glomerulonephritis
Urine culture	To evaluate for UTI
Urine calcium-to-creatinine ratio	To evaluate for hypercalciuria if hematuria persists for 1 year (urine calcium-creatinine ratio less than 0.2 is normal)
Renal ultrasound	Should be considered to evaluate for stones, tumors, hydronephrosis, structural anomalies, renal parenchymal dysplasia, medical renal disease, inflammation of the bladder, bladder polyps, and posterior urethral valves
Hearing test	If there is any reason to suspect familial renal disease

Suggested Work-Up of Isolated Asymptomatic Microscopic Hematuria

Urine culture	To evaluate for UTI
Serum creatinine	To evaluate for renal insufficiency
Renal ultrasound	Should be considered to evaluate for stones, tumors, hydronephrosis, structural anomalies, renal parenchymal dysplasia, medical renal disease, inflammation of the bladder, bladder polyps, and posterior urethral valves
Urine calcium-to-creatinine ratio	To evaluate for hypercalciuria if hematuria persists for 1 year (urine calcium/creatinine ratio less than 0.2 is normal)

Additional Work-Up of Isolated Asymptomatic Microscopic Hematuria

24-hour urine calcium excretion, serum electrolytes, calcium, phosphorus, magnesium

If hypercalciuria is identified

Coagulation studies

If an underlying coagulopathy is considered

Suggested Work-Up of Asymptomatic Microscopic Hematuria with Proteinuria

Quantification of urinary protein excretion with 24-hour collection or spot urine protein/creatinine ratio

To quantify urinary protein excretion

Serum creatinine and BUN, CBC, serum albumin, antistreptolysin O (ASO) titers streptozyme test, serum albumin, serum complement C3 and C4

To evaluate for glomerulonephritis

Antinuclear antibodies (ANA)

If lupus is suspected

Suggested Work-Up of Symptomatic Microscopic Hematuria

Serum creatinine and BUN, CBC, serum albumin, ASO titers, streptozyme test, serum albumin, serum complement C3 and C4

To evaluate for glomerulonephritis

ANA

To evaluate for lupus

Renal ultrasound or computed tomography (CT) scan

To evaluate for stones, tumors, hydronephrosis, structural anomalies, renal parenchymal dysplasia, medical renal disease, inflammation of the bladder, bladder polyps, and posterior urethral valves

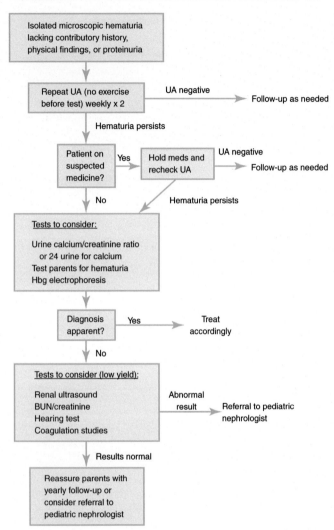

Figure 23-1. Evaluation of a child with asymptomatic microscopic hematuria.
(From Patel HP, Bissler JJ. Hematuria in children. *Pediatr Clin North Am* 2001;48:1519–1537, with permission.)

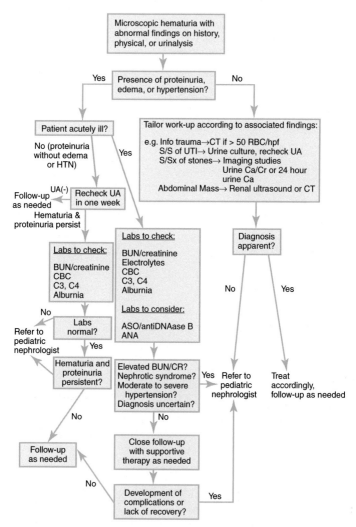

Figure 23-2. Evaluation of a child with microscopic hematuria associated with proteinuria, symptoms, or abnormalities in the history or physical examination.

(From Patel HP, Bissler JJ. Hematuria in children. *Pediatr Clin North Am* 2001;48:1519–1537, with permission.)

References

1. Gordon C, Stapleton FB. Hematuria in adolescents. *Adolesc Med* 2005;16:229–239.
2. Mahan JD, Turman MA, Mentser MI. Evaluation of hematuria, proteinuria, and hypertension in adolescents. *Pediatr Clin North Am* 1997;44:1573–1589.
3. Meyers KEC. Evaluation of hematuria in children. *Urol Clin North Am* 2004;31:559–573.
4. Pan CG. Evaluation of gross hematuria. *Pediatr Clin North Am* 2006;53:401–412.
5. Patel HP, Bissler JJ. Hematuria in children. *Pediatr Clin North Am* 2001;48:1519–1537.
6. Roy S. Hematuria. *Pediatr Rev* 1998;19:209–213.

Theodore X. O'Connell

The following discussion of hirsutism focuses on adolescent girls. For a discussion of hirsutism in infants or children, please see Chapter 35, Precocious Puberty.

Hirsutism is defined as the presence of excessive coarse terminal hair in a pattern not normal in females in areas such as the face, chest, or upper abdomen. This disorder is a sign of increased androgen action on hair follicles, which may result from increased levels of endogenous or exogenous androgens, or it may result from increased sensitivity of hair follicles to normal levels of circulating androgens. Hirsutism must be distinguished from *hypertrichosis,* which is the term used to describe the androgen-independent growth of hair that is vellus and does not follow the bodily distribution of the hair associated with male secondary sexual characteristics. Hypertrichosis may be familial or may be caused by medications or metabolic disorders.

Any patient who has either physical evidence of hirsutism or significant concern over excess hair growth should be evaluated. When evaluating hirsutism, it is important to determine whether hirsutism exists alone or whether virilization is also present. This distinction is important because virilization may reflect a serious underlying pathologic condition such as malignancy. Virilization manifests with a wide range of signs of androgen excess, such as acne, hirsutism, frontotemporal balding, amenorrhea, oligomenorrhea, deepening of the voice, and clitoromegaly.

The most common triggering factor for hirsutism is **excess androgen production**. Although androgens may come from an exogenous source, androgen excess is most commonly endogenous. The two primary sources of endogenous androgens are the adrenal glands and the ovaries. The most common cause of hyperandrogenism presenting in a teenage girl is **polycystic ovary syndrome (PCOS)**. The differential diagnosis also includes late-onset congential adrenal hyperplasia, virilizing tumors, Cushing syndrome, hyperprolactinemia, acromegaly, medications, and abnormalities of androgen action or metabolism.

A common endocrine disorder, PCOS affects 3% to 10% of premenopausal women. It represents a group of disorders associated with increased androgen production from the ovaries, adrenal glands, or both. The clinical presentation typically includes one or several of the following features: hirsutism, obesity, oligomenorrhea, anovulation, and infertility. At the 1990 National Institutes of Health (NIH) consensus conference, experts attempted to identify the key features needed to diagnose PCOS, noting the following as definite criteria: hyperandrogenism, menstrual dysfunction, clinical evidence of hyperandrogenism, and the exclusion of congenital adrenal hyperplasia. Probable criteria included insulin resistance, perimenarchal onset, an elevated ratio of luteinizing hormone (LH) to follicle stimulating hormone (FSH), and polycystic ovaries by sonography.

Patients with PCOS must be differentiated from individuals with variants of nonclassic congenital adrenal hyperplasia (CAH). The most common form of CAH is late-onset 21-hydroxylase deficiency. The diagnosis of nonclassic CAH can be made definitively by the use of adrenocorticotropin hormone (ACTH)-stimulation testing or can be inferred by measurement of early morning 17-hydroxyprogesterone levels.

Medications That May Cause Hirsutism

✓ Acetazolamide

✓ Anabolic steroids

✓ Cyclosporin

✓ Danazol

✓ Dilantin

✓ Methyldopa

✓ Metoclopramide

✓ Minoxidil

✓ Penicillamine

✓ Phenothiazines

✓ Progestins (especially levonorgestrel, norethindrone, and norgestrel)

✓ Reserpine

✓ Testosterone

Causes of Hirsutism

5-α-reductase deficiency

Adrenal hyperresponsiveness

Adrenal neoplasm

CAH

- 21-hydroxylase deficiency
- 11-hydroxylase deficiency
- 3-β-ol-dehydrogenase deficiency
- 12-ol-dehydrogenase deficiency
- Lipoid CAH

Congential anomalies

- Cornelia de Lange syndrome
- Hurler's syndrome
- Juvenile hypothyroidism
- Trisomy 18 (Edward syndrome)

Cushing's syndrome

Gonadal dysgenesis

Hyperprolactinemia

Idiopathic

Medications

Obesity (independent of PCOS)

Ovarian neoplasm

- Brenner's tumor
- Granulosa cell
- Gynandroblastoma
- Hypernephroma
- Lipoid cell
- Luteoma
- Sertoli-Leydig cell
- Thecoma

PCOS

Key Historical Features

✓ Onset and extent of hair growth

✓ Weight gain

✓ Abdominal symptoms

✓ Breast discharge or galactorrhea

✓ Skin symptoms such as acne, dryness, or striae

✓ Virilization symptoms

✓ Past medical history

✓ Menstrual and reproductive history

✓ Medications

✓ Family history

Key Physical Findings

✓ Blood pressure, height, weight

✓ Evaluation of hair distribution and characteristics

✓ Consider quantifying degree of hirsutism using the Ferriman and Gallwey scoring system

✓ Skin evaluation (for acanthosis nigricans, acne, striae, hyperpigmentation)

✓ Breast examination for nipple discharge or galactorrhea

✓ Abdominal examination for masses

✓ Pelvic examination for masses

✓ Signs of Cushing syndrome

✓ Signs of virilization

Suggested Work-Up

Serum testosterone and DHEA sulfate (DHEA-S)	To evaluate for ovarian and adrenal tumors. Total testosterone levels >1.5 ng/mL or DHEA-S levels >700 μg/dL are suggestive of androgen-producing neoplasms
Serum 17α-hydroxyprogesterone (17-OHP)	To evaluate for late-onset adrenal hyperplasia
	<200 ng/dL is unlikely to be 21-hydroxylase deficiency
	200–400 ng/dL indicates low likelihood 21-hydroxylase deficiency, but ACTH stimulation test recommended
	400–1000 ng/dL is suggestive of 21-hydroxylase deficiency and ACTH stimulation test is recommended
	>1000 ng/dL is diagnostic of 21-hydroxylase deficiency
Serum prolactin	To evaluate for pituitary tumors

Thyroid-stimulating hormone (TSH)	To evaluate for thyroid dysfunction
Fasting serum glucose	To evaluate for insulin resistance in patients suspected of having PCOS

Additional Work-Up

ACTH stimulation test with measurement of 17-OHP at baseline and 60 minutes after administration of 0.25 mg cosyntropin	When CAH is suspected. In 21-hydroxylase deficiency, an increase of 17-OHP to more than 1500 ng/dL at 60 minutes is usually seen.
LH and FSH	May be useful in confirming the diagnosis of PCOS. Elevated LH level is suggestive of PCOS, particularly when the LH-FSH ratio exceeds 2.5.
24-hour urinary collection for free cortisol and creatinine levels	If Cushing syndrome is suspected
Dexamethasone suppression test (1 mg dexamethasone at 11 PM with 8 AM serum cortisol levels measured the next day)	If urinary free cortisol level is elevated. The morning cortisol level should be less than 5.0 µg/dL after the dexamethasone dosing.
Glucose tolerance test	In patients with suspected PCOS with elevated fasting serum glucose
Computed tomography (CT) of the abdomen and pelvis	To assess the adrenal glands and ovaries in patients whose history, physical examination, or laboratory evaluation suggest the presence of a virilizing tumor

References

1. Bailey-Pridham DD, Sanfilippo JS. Hirsutism in the adolescent female. *Pediatr Clin North Am* 1989;36:581–599.
2. Bates GW. Hirsutism and androgen excess in childhood and adolescence. *Pediatr Clin North Am* 1981;28:513–530.
3. Gilchrist VJ, Hecht BR. A practical approach to hirsutism. *Am Fam Physician* 1995;52: 1837–1846.
4. Gordon CM. Menstrual disorders in adolescents: excess androgens and the polycystic ovary syndrome. *Pediatr Clin North Am* 1999;46:519–543.

5. Hunter MH, Carek PJ. Evaluation and treatment of women with hirsutism. *Am Fam Physician* 2003;67:2565–2572.

6. Leung AK, Robson WL. Hirsutism. *Int J Dermatol* 1993;32:773–777.

7. Miller WL. Pathophysiology, genetics, and treatment of hyperandrogenism. *Pediatr Clin North Am* 1997;44:375–395.

8. Plouffe L. Disorders of excessive hair growth in the adolescent. *Obstet Gynecol Clin* 2000;27:79–99.

9. Redmond GP, Bergfeld WF. Diagnostic approach to adrogen disorders in women: acne, hirsutism, and alopecia. *Cleve Clin J Med* 1990;57:423–427.

10. Rosenfield RL. Hyperandrogenism in peripubertal girls. *Pediatr Clin North Am* 1990;37:1333–1358.

11. Speroff L, Glass RH, Kase NG. *Clinical Gynecologic Endocrinology and Infertility*, 6th ed. Baltimore: Lippincott Williams & Wilkins; 1999:529–556.

Jonathan M. Wong and Theodore X. O'Connell

This discussion focuses on neonatal hyperbilirubinemia in infants 35 or more weeks of gestation.

Neonatal hyperbilirubinemia is defined as a total serum bilirubin greater than 5 mg/dL. Jaundice results from the deposition of unconjugated bilirubin pigment in the skin and mucus membranes. Up to 60% of term newborns have clinical jaundice in the first week of life, yet few have significant underlying disease. However, neonatal hyperbilirubinemia can be associated with hemolytic disease, metabolic and endocrine disorders, infections, and anatomic abnormalities of the liver.

Bilirubin is the final product of heme degradation. Newborns produce bilirubin at twice the rate of adults because of relative polycythemia and increased red blood cell (RBC) turnover. Bilirubin production typically declines to adult levels within 10-14 days after birth. Neonatal hyperbilirubinemia results from a predisposition to the production in newborn infants and their limited ability to excrete it.

The term *kernicterus* has come to be used interchangeably with both the acute and chronic findings of bilirubin encephalopathy. Bilirubin encephalopathy describes the clinical central nervous system (CNS) findings caused by bilirubin toxicity to the basal ganglia and various brainstem nuclei. It is unclear what level of total serum bilirubin is associated with kernicterus, although most experts agree that bilirubin levels greater than 20 mg/dL in the term infant warrant concern. Early signs of kernicterus are subtle and nonspecific, but bilirubin encephalopathy may be more evident by 3 years of age and leads to developmental and motor delays, sensorineural deafness, and mild mental retardation.

Physiologic jaundice in the healthy term newborn usually peaks at 5 to 6 mg/dL on the third to fourth day of life and then declines over the first week after birth. Bilirubin elevations up to 12 mg/dL can sometimes occur. Infants with multiple risk factors may develop an exaggerated form of physiologic jaundice. Breastfed newborns may be at increased risk for exaggerated physiologic jaundice because of relative caloric deprivation and mild dehydration with resulting delayed passage of meconium in the first few days of life. Formula supplementation may be necessary, but breastfeeding should be continued to maintain breast milk production. Serum bilirubin concentrations higher than 17 mg/dL in full-term infants are no longer considered physiologic, and a cause of pathologic jaundice can usually be identified in these infants.

Breast milk jaundice occurs later in the newborn period, with the bilirubin level usually peaking between 6 and 14 days of life. Breast milk jaundice may occur in up to one third of healthy breastfed infants and is believed to be the result of substances in maternal milk which may inhibit normal bilirubin metabolism. The bilirubin level usually falls after the infant is 2 weeks old but may remain elevated for 1 to 3 months. Breastfeeding may be temporarily interrupted if the diagnosis of breast milk jaundice is in doubt or the total serum bilirubin level becomes markedly elevated.

Any jaundice beyond physiologic and breast milk jaundice is considered pathologic. Features of pathologic jaundice include the appearance of jaundice within 24 hours after birth, an increase of total serum bilirubin greater than 5 mg/dL per day, and a total serum bilirubin level higher than 17 mg/dL in a full-term newborn. Other features suggesting pathologic jaundice include prolonged jaundice, evidence of underlying illness, and elevation of the serum conjugated bilirubin to greater than 2 mg/dL or more than 20% of the total serum bilirubin concentration.

Risk factors for neonatal hyperbilirubinemia are outlined below.

Medications Associated with Hyperbilirubinemia

- Acetaminophen
- Aspirin
- Chloramphenicol
- Corticosteroids
- Diazepam (maternal use)
- Erythromycin
- Pitocin (maternal use)
- Rifampin
- Streptomycin
- Sulfa
- Sulfisoxazole acetyl with erythromycin ethylsuccinate
- Tetracycline

Causes of Hyperbilirubinemia

Increased Bilirubin Load

Hemolytic Causes (increased unconjugated bilirubin level, >6% reticulocytes, hemoglobin concentration of <13 g/dL)

- Positive Coombs' test
  - o Rh factor incompatibility
  - o ABO incompatibility
  - o Minor antigens
- Negative Coombs' test
  - o Drugs
  - o Elliptocytosis

- o Glucose-6-phosphate dehydrogenase (G6PD) deficiency
- o Hemoglobinopathies
- o Pyruvate kinase deficiency
- o Sepsis
- o Spherocytosis

Nonhemolytic causes (increased unconjugated bilirubin level, normal percentage of reticulocytes)

- • Exaggerated enterohepatic circulation
  - o Breast milk jaundice
  - o Cystic fibrosis
  - o Hirschsprung disease
  - o Ileal atresia
  - o Pyloric stenosis
- • Extravascular sources
  - o Bruising
  - o CNS hemorrhage
  - o Cephalohematoma
  - o Swallowed blood
- • Polycythemia
  - o Delayed cord clamping
  - o Fetal-maternal transfusion
  - o Twin-twin transfusion

Decreased Bilirubin Conjugation

Characterized by increased unconjugated bilirubin level, normal percentage of reticulocytes

- • Breast milk jaundice
- • Crigler-Najjar syndrome types 1 and 2
- • Gilbert syndrome
- • Hypothyroidism
- • Physiologic jaundice

Impaired Bilirubin Excretion

Characterized by increased unconjugated and conjugated bilirubin levels, negative Coombs' test, conjugated bilirubin level greater than 2 mg/dL or more than 20% of total serum bilirubin level, and conjugated bilirubin in the urine

- • Biliary obstruction
  - o Biliary atresia

- o Choledochal cyst
- o Dubin-Johnson syndrome
- o Gallstones
- o Neoplasm
- o Primary sclerosing cholangitis
- o Rotor syndrome
- Chromosomal abnormality
  - o Trisomy 18
  - o Trisomy 21
  - o Turner syndrome
- Infection
  - o Hepatitis
  - o Herpes simplex
  - o Rubella
  - o Sepsis
  - o Syphilis
  - o Toxoplasmosis
  - o Tuberculosis
  - o Urinary tract infection (UTI)
- Medications
  - o Acetaminophen
  - o Alcohol
  - o Aspirin
  - o Corticosteroids
  - o Erythromycin
  - o Rifampin
  - o Sulfa
  - o Tetracycline
- Metabolic disorder
  - o α_1-antitrypsin deficiency
  - o Cystic fibrosis
  - o Galactosemia
  - o Gaucher disease
  - o Glycogen storage disease
  - o Hypothyroidism
  - o Niemann-Pick disease
  - o Wilson disease

Key Historical Features

Risk Factors for Hyperbilirubinemia in Newborns

Maternal factors

✓ Blood type ABO or Rh incompatibility

✓ Ethnicity (Asian, Native American)

✓ Exclusive breastfeeding, particularly if nursing is not going well and weight loss is excessive

✓ Medications (see page 172)

✓ Maternal age > 25 years

Neonatal factors

✓ Birth trauma (cephalohematoma, cutaneous bruising, instrumented delivery)

✓ Excessive weight loss after birth

✓ Gestational age (age 35-36 weeks is a major risk factor; age 37-38 weeks is a minor risk factor)

✓ Infections: toxoplasmosis, other agents, rubella, cytomegalovirus, herpes simplex (TORCH)

✓ Jaundice observed before hospital discharge

✓ Macrosomic infant of a diabetic mother

✓ Male gender

✓ Medications (see page 172)

✓ Polycythemia

✓ Previous sibling with hyperbilirubinemia

Key Physical Findings

✓ Weight measurement with comparison to birth weight

✓ General examination for evidence of infection

✓ Evaluation for dehydration

✓ Skin examination for jaundice, pallor, petechiae, extravasated blood, or excessive bruising

✓ Abdominal examination for hepatosplenomegaly

Suggested Work-Up

The suggested work-up for the jaundiced infant of 35 or more weeks' gestation depends on the clinical picture and is outlined below.

A transcutaneous bilirubin or total serum bilirubin measurement, or both, should be performed on every infant who is jaundiced in the first 24 hours after birth and in all infants in whom jaundice appears excessive for the infant's age. If there is any doubt about the degree of jaundice, the transcutaneous bilirubin or total serum bilirubin should be measured. All bilirubin levels should be interpreted on a nomogram according to the infant's age in hours (Figures 25-1 and 25-2). An algorithm for the management of jaundice is presented in Figure 25-3.

Jaundice in the First 24 Hours

Measurement of transcutaneous bilirubin and/or total serum bilirubin	To determine bilirubin level and interpret on a nomogram according to the infant's age in hours

Jaundice Appears Excessive for Infant's Age

Measurement of transcutaneous bilirubin and/or total serum bilirubin	To determine bilirubin level and interpret on a nomogram according to the infant's age in hours

Infant Receiving Phototherapy or Total Serum Bilirubin is Rising Rapidly and Unexplained by History and Physical Examination

Blood type and Coombs' test if not obtained with cord blood	To evaluate for isoimmune hemolysis
Complete blood count (CBC) and smear	To evaluate for infection, evidence of hemolysis, or polycythemia
Direct (conjugated) bilirubin	To evaluate for causes of impaired bilirubin excretion

Consider:

Reticulocyte count	To evaluate for hemolysis
G6PD assay	To evaluate for G6PD deficiency in infants whose family history or ethnic or geographic origin suggest the likelihood of G6PD deficiency
End Tidal CO (ETCO) if available	To evaluate for hemolysis
Repeat total serum bilirubin in 4 to 24 hours depending on infant's age and total serum bilirubin level	

Total Serum Bilirubin Concentration Approaching Exchange Levels or Responding to Phototherapy

Reticulocyte count	To evaluate for hemolysis
G6PD assay	To evaluate for G6PD deficiency
Albumin	To evaluate for hypoalbuminemia
ETCO if available	To evaluate for hemolysis

Elevated Direct (Conjugated) Bilirubin Level

Urinalysis and urine culture Evaluate for sepsis if indicated by history and physical examination	To evaluate for UTI

Jaundice Present at or Beyond Age 3 Weeks, or Sick Infant

Total and direct (conjugated) bilirubin level	To determine bilirubin level and evaluate for cholestasis
Check results of newborn thyroid and galactosemia screen	To evaluate for hypothyroidism and galactosemia

Additional Work-Up

Peripheral blood smear	If hemolysis is suspected
Red cell enzyme studies	If G6PD deficiency or pyruvate kinase deficiency is suspected
Hemoglobin electrophoresis	If hemoglobinopathy is suspected
Thyroid-stimulating hormong (TSH)	If hypothyroidism is suspected
Toxicology screen	If the history is suggestive of toxin exposure
Purified protein derivative (PPD)	If tuberculosis infection is suspected
Toxoplasmosis titers	If toxoplasmosis is suspected
Syphilis titers	If syphilis is suspected
Chromosomal analysis	If a chromosomal abnormality is suspected

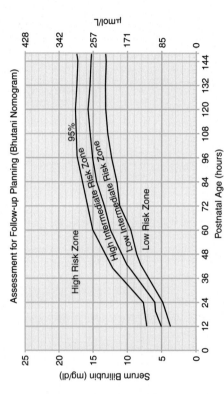

Figure 25-1. Bilirubin levels and risk of significant hyperbilirubinemia. Nomogram for designation of risk in 2840 well newborns of ≥36 weeks' gestational age with birth weight of 2000 g or more or ≥35 weeks' gestational age and birth weight of 2500 g or more based on the hour-specific serum bilirubin values. The serum bilirubin level was obtained before discharge, and the zone in which the value fell predicted the likelihood of a subsequent bilirubin level exceeding the 95th percentile (high-risk zone). This nomogram should not be used to represent the natural history of neonatal hyperbilirubinemia.

(From Bhutani VK, Johnson L, Sivieri EM. Predictive ability of a predischarge hour-specific serum bilirubin for subsequent significant hyperbilirubinemia in healthy term and near-term newborns. *Pediatrics* 1999;103:6–14, with permission.)

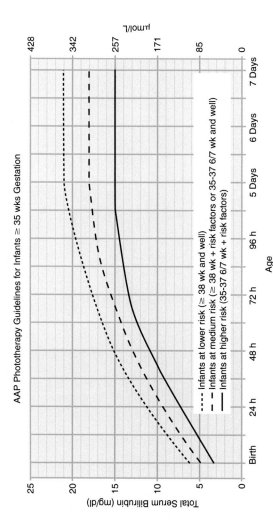

Figure 25-2. AAP Phototherapy Guidelines for Infants ≥35 weeks' gestation.
(From Subcommittee on Hyperbilirubinemia, American Academy of Pediatrics. Management of hyperbilirubinemia in the newborn infant 35 or more weeks of gestation. *Pediatrics* 2004;114:297–316, with permission.)

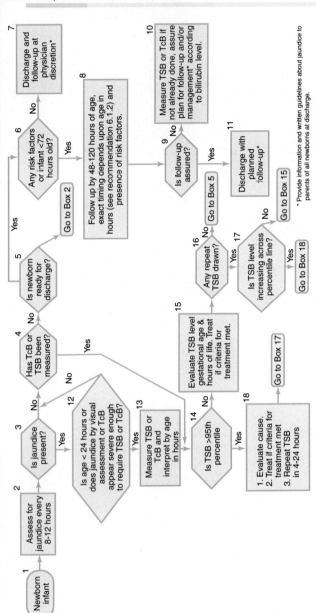

Figure 25-3. Algorithm for the management of jaundice in the newborn nursery.
(From Subcommittee on Hyperbilirubinemia, American Academy of Pediatrics. Management of hyperbilirubinemia in the newborn infant of ≥35 weeks' of gestation. *Pediatrics* 2004;114:297–316, with permission.)

References

1. Bhutani VK, Johnson L, Sivieri EM. Predictive ability of a predischarge hour-specific serum bilirubin for subsequent significant hyperbilirubinemia in healthy term and near-term newborns. *Pediatrics* 1999;103:6–14.
2. Dennery PA, Seidman DS, Stevenson DK. Neonatal hyperbilirubinemia. *N Engl J Med* 2001;344:581–590.
3. Porter ML, Dennis BL. Hyperbilirubinemia in the term newborn. *Am Fam Physician* 2002;65:599–606.
4. Subcommittee on Hyperbilirubinemia. American Academy of Pediatrics. Management of hyperbilirubinemia in the newborn infant 35 or more weeks of gestation. *Pediatrics* 2004;114:297–316.

Theodore X. O'Connell

The overall incidence of venous thrombotic events (TE) in children is estimated to be between 0.7 and 1.9 per 100,000 children. Newborns are at particularly high risk of TE, presumably because of their immature coagulation system marked by decreased activity of anticoagulant factors, including antithrombin, protein C, and protein S.

Hypercoagulable conditions are classified as *primary,* an inherited condition, or *secondary,* an acquired state. The inherited disorders include factor V Leiden; prothrombin G20210A gene mutation; hyperhomocysteinemia; dysfibrinogenemia; elevated factor VIII level; and deficiencies of antithrombin, protein C, and protein S. Acquired hypercoagulable conditions include the antiphospholipid syndrome (lupus anticoagulant and anticardiolipin antibody); hyperhomocysteinemia; and the commonly known thrombosis risk factors of pregnancy, cancer, and estrogen-containing medications.

Until recently, the assessment and management of children with thromboembolism have relied almost exclusively on data from the adult experience with thrombosis. Developmental differences in the coagulation system of children and differences in medical problems underlying the development of thrombosis in children are now being considered in the management of pediatric thrombosis.

Most case of TE within the first year of life are associated with central venous access devices. In addition, spontaneous thromboses in the renal, caval, portal, or hepatic venous systems have been reported in neonates. These TE often are associated with acquired predisposing factors such as sepsis, peripartum asphyxia, dehydration, or maternal diabetes. By 6 months of age, infants' levels of almost all of the coagulation factors reach adult values, and the risk of thrombosis decreases. TEs after infancy are more often multifactorial and associated with other medical conditions, outlined below.

Inherited prothrombotic disorders are usually suspected in children with an unexplained cause for thrombosis, a positive family history of thrombosis, a history of recurrent TE, or thromboses in an unusual location. The most common inherited prothrombotic disorders are due to mutations in the factor V Leiden gene or prothrombin gene, followed by deficiencies of antithrombin (AT), protein C, and protein S. Hyperhomocysteinemia and dysfibrinogenemia are also among the more common causes of thrombosis. The relative risk of recurrent TE increases with the number of inherited susceptibility genes.

No standardized approach to screening patients for hypercoagulability has been established. The cost-effectiveness of performing the laboratory examination is unknown, and the work-up typically is expensive. Most clinicians take into consideration patient risk factors when deciding on the need for an extensive work-up. A work-up should be considered when there is an unexplained cause for thrombosis, a positive family history of thrombosis, a history of recurrent TE, or thromboses in an unusual location.

Risk Factors for Venous Thrombosis

Activated Protein C Resistance or Protein C Concentrate Administration

Autoimmune Disorders

- Antiphospholipid antibody syndrome
- Behçet's disease
- Diabetes mellitus
- Inflammatory bowel disease
- Lupus anticoagulant

Chemotherapy (L-asparaginase, prednisone)

Congenital heart disease

Dehydration

Immobilization

Indwelling catheter device

Infection

- HIV
- Suppurative thrombophlebitis
- Varicella

Inherited or acquired thrombophilias

Leg paralysis

Liver disease

Malignancy

Oral contraceptive and other estrogen use

Polycythemia

Pregnancy

Previous venous thromboembolism

Renal disease (chronic renal disease, nephrotic syndrome)

Sickle cell disease

Surgical and nonsurgical trauma

Thalassemia (postsplenectomy portal vein thrombosis)

Suggested Work-Up

✓ Anticardiolipin antibody

✓ Anti-thrombin III

✓ Factor V Leiden

✓ Factor VIII level

✓ Fibrinogen (including immunologic/functional studies and thrombin time)

✓ Homocysteine level

✓ Lipoprotein(a)

✓ Lupus anticoagulant

✓ Protein C

✓ Protein S

✓ Prothrombin G20210A

Additional Work-Up (Studies for Rare Causes of Thrombosis)

✓ Activated protein C resistance

✓ Factor XI

✓ Factor XII

✓ Heparin cofactor 2

✓ Thrombomodulin

✓ Tissue factor pathway inhibitor

✓ Plasminogen

✓ Plasminogen activator inhibitor-1

✓ Tissue plasminogen activator

References

1. Alpert MA. Homocysteine, atherosclerosis, and thrombosis. *South Med J* 1999;92:858–865.
2. Barger AP, Hurley R. Evaluation of the hypercoagulable state: whom to screen, how to test and treat. *Postgrad Med* 2000;108:59–66.
3. DeStefano V, Finazzi G, Mannucci PM. Inherited thrombophilia: pathogenesis, clinical syndromes, and management. *Blood* 1996;87:531.
4. Faioni EM, et al. Free protein S deficiency is risk factor for venous thrombosis. *Thromb Haimost* 1997;78:1343.
5. Federman DG, Kirsner RS. An update on hypercoagulable disorders. *Arch Intern Med* 2001;161:1051–1056.
6. Hoppe C, Matsunaga A. Pediatric thrombosis. *Pediatr Clin North Am* 2002;49:1257–1283.
7. Koster T, et al. Role of clotting factor VIII in effect of von Willebrand factor on occurrence of deep-vein thrombosis. *Lancet* 1995;345:152–155.

8. Poort SR, et al. A common genetic variant in the 3'-untranslated region of the prothrombin gene is asscociated with elevated plasma prothrombin levels and an increase in thrombosis. *Thromb Haimost* 1997;78:1430–1433.
9. Tait RC, et al. Prevalence of protein C deficiency in the healthy population. *Thomb Haimost* 1995;73:87.

Kevin Haggerty

The relevance of childhood blood pressure (BP) measurement to pediatric health care and the development of adult essential hypertension has undergone substantial conceptual change during the past two decades. Hypertension and its sequelae traditionally have been considered a disease acquired in middle age, but hypertension often begins in childhood and adolescence. It is now understood that hypertension detected in some children may be a sign of an underlying disease, such as renal parenchymal disease, whereas in other cases the elevated BP may represent the early onset of essential hypertension. The awareness of pediatric hypertension among the medical community and general public has increased in recent years, leading to increasing numbers of hypertensive children coming to medical attention. Hypertension present in childhood predisposes the patient to cerebrovascular disease, left ventricular hypertrophy, atherosclerosis, coronary artery disease, and retinal changes.

The most commonly used definitions of normal and abnormal BP in childhood come from the National High Blood Pressure Education Program Working Group. These definitions are endorsed in the Seventh Report of the Joint National Committee on Prevention, Detection, Evaluation, and Treatment of High Blood Pressure (JNC 7). *Normal* BP is defined as systolic and diastolic BP less than the 90th percentile for age and sex. *High-normal* BP is defined as average systolic or diastolic BP greater than or equal to the 90th percentile but less than the 95th percentile. *Hypertension* is defined as average systolic or diastolic readings greater than the 95th percentile based on age, gender, and height percentile (Tables 27-1 and 27-2). At least three abnormal readings, obtained on separate occasions over a period of several weeks, should be obtained before entertaining a diagnosis of hypertension in an individual patient. A separate set of BP percentile curves has been established for infants aged 0 to 12 months (Figures 27-1 and 27-2).

The causes of hypertension in children are diverse, with a significantly greater percentage of hypertensive children having secondary forms of hypertension compared with adults. In children, most causes of secondary hypertension are renal in origin. **Essential (primary) hypertension** becomes more prevalent with increasing age to the point that most older adolescents with hypertension have the primary form.

BP in childhood may predict adult BP. The Muscatine study demonstrated subjects with diastolic BP, above the 90th percentile in childhood to be twice as likely to develop adult hypertension than expected. In addition, the likelihood of developing adult hypertension increased with increasing numbers of childhood readings above the 90th percentile.

The absence of abnormal readings in childhood was associated with a reduced risk of developing adult hypertension. Although a single elevated blood pressure measurement in childhood does not necessarily predict the future development of hypertension, such a child should be monitored more closely. In addition, the child should be monitored for the presence of other cardiovascular risk factors, such as hyperlipidemia.

Current recommendations are for all children 3 and older to have blood pressure measured with every visit to their health care provider. Children under 3 with risk factors such as low birth weight, extended stay in the neonatal intensive care unit (NICU), cardiac abnormalities, recurrent urinary tract infections (UTIs), known or family history of renal disease, or solid organ transplants should have BP measurements with each clinical visit.

A conventional mercury column or aneroid sphygmomanometer is recommended, although an automated oscillometric device may be used in infants and toddlers who will not cooperate with manual BP measurement. The bladder of the cuff should encircle 80% to 100% of the circumference of the upper arm, and its width should be at least 40% of the upper arm circumference. The disappearance of the 5th Karotkoff sound is used to define the diastolic BP.

Medications and Substances Associated with Hypertension

- Albuterol
- Anabolic steroids
- Caffeine
- Cocaine
- Ephedrine
- Glucocorticoids
- Methamphetamine
- Pseudoephederine
- Ritalin
- Sumatriptan
- Theophyilline

Causes of Hypertension

Primary (Essential) Hypertension

Secondary Hypertension

Infants aged 0 to 12 months
- Bronchopulmonary dysplasia
- Coarctation of the aorta
- Congenital renal disease

- Intraventricular hemorrhage
- Patent ductus arteriosus
- Renal vein thrombosis

Children and adolescents

- Coarctation of the aorta
- Congenital adrenal hyperplasia
- Hyperthyroidism
- Liddle syndrome
- Mineral corticoid excess
- Neoplasm
- Neurofibromatosis
- Pheochromocytoma
- Renal disease
  - o Glomerulonephritis
  - o Reflux nephropathy
  - o Renal artery stenosis
  - o Renal venous thrombosis
  - o Structural renal disease
  - o Wilms or neurogenic tumors
- Sleep apnea
- Systemic lupus erythematosus
- Turner's syndrome
- Williams syndrome

Key Historical Features

Symptoms Suggestive of Hypertension

- Diplopia
- Dizziness
- Epistaxis
- Headaches
- Vomiting

Symptoms Suggestive of Underlying Renal Disease

- Edema
- Enuresis
- Fatigue
- Gross hematuria

Sympotms Suggestive of Heart Disease
- Chest pain
- Exertional dyspnea
- Palpitations

Medical History
- Chronic illnesses
- Neonatal history of umbilical line placement (important in infants with hypertension)
- Prior hospitalizations
- Recurrent UTIs
- Trauma
- Unexplained fevers

Medications (Prescription and Over-the-Counter)

Family History
- Cardiovascular disease
- Diabetes
- Hyperlipidemia
- Hypertension
- Renal disease
- Stroke

Surgical History

Social History
- Alcohol use
- Illicit drug use
- Tobacco use

Key Physical Findings

✓ Height and weight percentiles

✓ Vital signs with systolic and diastolic BPs matched against standards for age, sex, height (see Tables 27-1 and 27-2). Consider measuring the BP in all four extremities regardless of the child's age to evaluate for coarctation of the aorta

✓ Funduscopic examination to evaluate for microvascular changes, pinpoint hemorrhages, and "cotton wool" spots

✓ Head and neck examination to evaluate for moon facies, suggestive of Cushing syndrome; a webbed-neck, suggestive of Turner syndrome; or tonsillar hypertrophy, which may result in obstructive sleep apnea. The thyroid should be palpated for thyromegaly

✓ Cardiovascular examination for tachycardia, murmur, friction rub, or apical heave

✓ Pulmonary examination

✓ Abdominal examination for a palpable mass or abdominal bruit

✓ Genital examination for ambiguous genitalia

✓ Skin examination for flushing or diaphoresis suggestive of pheochromocytoma, café au lait spots suggestive of neurofibromatosis, malar rash suggestive of lupus, or acanthosis nigracans suggestive of diabetes

Initial Work-Up

Many hypertensive children will have otherwise normal physical examinations, even in the presence of significant underlying renal or other organ system disease. Therefore, laboratory testing is usually necessary to complete the child's evaluation. The child's age, history, physical examination findings, and degree of BP elevation should be used to decide what are the most appropriate studies for a particular child. All hypertensive children should undergo the following screening laboratory tests:

- Urinalysis and culture
- Electrolytes, blood urea nitrogen (BUN), creatinine
- Glucose
- Calcium
- Phosphorus
- Uric acid
- Lipid panel
- Complete blood count (CBC) with differential and platelet count
- Echocardiogram in all hypertensive children is suggested by some authorities because left ventricular hypertrophy can be present even in children with mild hypertension.
- Referral to a pediatric ophthalmologist for a thorough retinal examination may be considered in children with hypertension, particularly if the echocardiogram is abnormal.

Additional Work-Up

Specific laboratory tests (as indicated by the history, physical examination, and screening tests):

24-hour urine collection for protein excretion and creatinine clearance	If renal disease is suspected or determined by the screening tests

Urine and serum catecholamines	If pheochromocytoma is suspected
Serum cortisol level	If Cushing's syndrome is suspected
Thyroid-stimulating hormone (TSH), thyroxine (T_4), tri-iodothyronine (T_3)	If a thyroid disorder is suspected
Echocardiogram	If cardiac disease is suspected on the basis of a murmur or other abnormal finding on physical examination. An echocardiogram for all hypertensive children is suggested by some authorities because left ventricular hypertrophy can be present even in children with mild hypertension.
Serum 17α-hydroxyprogesterone	If congenital adrenal hyperplasia is suspected
Plasma aldosterone	If hyperaldosteronism is suspected
Renal ultrasound	If renal disease is suspected to evaluate the contour and texture of the kidneys and to screen for gross renal abnormalities
Computed tomography (CT) scan of abdomen and pelvis	If an abdominal mass is palpated on physical examination to evaluate for the presence of tumor

Specialized studies (typically performed at referral centers or by pediatric subspecialists in the evaluation of pediatric hypertension):

Plasma rennin and 24-hour urinary sodium excretion	To evaluate for renal artery stenosis
Renal ultrasound with Doppler study of renal arteries	To evaluate for renal artery stenosis
Captopril challenge test	To evaluate for renal artery stenosis
Renal angiography with renal vein renins	To evaluate for renal artery stenosis

Magnetic resonance angiography	To evaluate for renal artery stenosis
Captopril renal scan	To evaluate for renal artery stenosis
Ambulatory BP monitoring	Not yet endorsed by consensus bodies for routine use in children, but may affect the management of childhood hypertension and may predict the presence of secondary hypertension
Renal biopsy	To establish a tissue diagnosis in renal disease
Angiography	To evaluate for renal artery stenosis

Age, yr	Blood Pressure Percentile*	Systolic Blood Pressure by Percentile of Height, mm Hg⁺							Diastolic Blood Pressure by Percentile of Height, mm Hg⁺						
		5%	10%	25%	50%	75%	90%	95%	5%	10%	25%	50%	75%	90%	95%
1	90th	94	95	97	98	100	102	102	50	51	52	53	54	54	55
	95th	98	99	101	102	104	106	106	55	55	56	57	58	59	59
2	90th	98	99	100	102	104	105	106	55	55	56	57	58	59	59
	95th	101	102	104	106	108	109	110	59	59	60	61	62	63	63
3	90th	100	101	103	105	107	108	109	59	59	60	61	62	63	63
	95th	104	105	107	109	111	112	113	63	63	64	65	66	67	67
4	90th	102	103	105	107	109	110	111	62	62	63	64	65	66	66
	95th	106	107	109	111	113	114	115	66	67	67	68	69	70	71
5	90th	104	105	106	108	110	111	112	65	65	66	67	68	69	69
	95th	108	109	110	112	114	115	116	69	70	70	71	72	73	74
6	90th	105	106	108	110	111	113	114	67	68	69	70	70	71	72
	95th	109	110	112	114	115	117	117	72	72	73	74	75	76	76
7	90th	106	107	109	111	113	114	115	69	70	71	72	72	73	74
	95th	110	111	113	115	116	118	119	74	74	75	76	77	78	78
8	90th	107	108	110	112	114	115	116	71	71	72	73	74	75	75
	95th	111	112	114	116	118	119	120	75	76	76	77	78	79	80
9	90th	109	110	112	113	115	117	117	72	73	73	74	75	76	77
	95th	113	114	116	117	119	121	121	76	77	78	79	80	80	81
10	90th	110	112	113	115	117	118	119	73	74	74	75	76	77	77
	95th	114	115	117	119	121	122	123	77	78	79	80	80	81	81
11	90th	112	113	115	117	119	120	121	74	74	75	76	77	78	78
	95th	116	117	119	121	123	124	125	78	79	79	80	81	82	83

Table 27-1. 90th and 95th Percentile Blood Pressures for Boys Aged 1 to 17 Years by Height Percentile

Continued

Age, yr	Blood Pressure Percentile*	Systolic Blood Pressure by Percentile of Height, mm Hg†							Diastolic Blood Pressure by Percentile of Height, mm Hg†						
		5%	10%	25%	50%	75%	90%	95%	5%	10%	25%	50%	75%	90%	95%
12	90th	115	116	117	119	121	123	123	75	75	76	77	78	78	79
	95th	119	120	121	123	125	126	127	79	79	80	81	82	83	83
13	90th	117	118	120	122	124	125	126	75	76	76	77	78	79	79
	95th	121	122	124	126	128	129	130	79	80	81	82	83	83	84
14	90th	120	121	123	125	126	128	128	76	76	77	78	79	80	80
	95th	124	125	127	128	130	132	132	80	81	81	82	83	84	85
15	90th	123	124	125	127	129	131	131	77	77	78	79	80	81	81
	95th	127	128	129	131	133	134	135	81	82	83	83	84	85	86
16	90th	125	126	128	130	132	133	134	79	79	80	81	82	82	83
	95th	129	130	132	134	136	137	138	83	83	84	85	86	87	87
17	90th	128	129	131	133	134	136	136	81	81	82	83	84	85	85
	95th	132	133	135	136	138	140	140	85	85	86	87	88	89	89

*Blood pressure percentile was determined by a single measurement.

†Height percentile was determined by standard growth curves.

(From Update on the 1987 Task Force Report on High Blood Pressure in Children and Adolescents: A Working Group Report from the National High Blood Pressure Education Program. *Pediatrics* 1996;98:649–658, with permission.)

Table 27-1. 90th and 95th Percentile Blood Pressures for Boys Aged 1 to 17 Years by Height Percentile

	Blood Pressure Percentile*	Systolic Blood Pressure by Percentile of Height, mm Hg+							Diastolic Blood Pressure by Percentile of Height, mm Hg+						
Age, yr		5%	10%	25%	50%	75%	90%	95%	5%	10%	25%	50%	75%	90%	95%
1	90th	97	98	99	100	102	103	104	53	53	53	54	55	56	56
	95th	101	102	103	104	105	107	107	57	57	57	58	59	60	60
2	90th	99	99	100	102	103	104	105	57	57	58	58	59	60	61
	95th	102	103	104	105	107	108	109	61	61	62	62	63	64	65
3	90th	100	100	102	103	104	105	106	61	61	61	62	63	63	64
	95th	104	104	105	107	108	109	110	65	65	65	66	67	67	68
4	90th	101	102	103	104	106	107	108	63	63	64	65	65	66	67
	95th	105	106	107	108	109	111	111	67	67	68	69	69	70	71
5	90th	103	103	104	106	107	108	109	65	66	66	67	68	68	69
	95th	107	107	108	110	111	112	113	69	70	70	71	72	72	73
6	90th	104	105	106	107	109	110	111	67	67	68	69	69	70	71
	95th	108	109	110	111	112	114	114	71	71	72	73	73	74	75
7	90th	106	107	108	109	110	112	112	69	69	69	70	71	72	72
	95th	110	110	112	113	114	115	116	73	73	73	74	75	76	76
8	90th	108	109	110	111	112	113	114	70	70	71	71	72	73	74
	95th	112	112	113	115	116	117	118	74	74	75	75	76	77	78
9	90th	110	110	112	113	114	115	116	71	72	72	73	74	74	75
	95th	114	114	115	117	118	119	120	75	76	76	77	78	78	79
10	90th	112	112	114	115	116	117	118	73	73	73	74	75	76	76
	95th	116	116	117	119	120	121	122	77	77	77	78	79	80	80
11	90th	114	114	116	117	118	119	120	74	74	75	75	76	77	77
	95th	118	118	119	121	122	123	124	78	78	79	79	80	81	81

Continued

Table 27-2. 90th and 95th Percentile Blood Pressures for Girls Aged 1 to 17 Years by Height Percentile.

Age, yr	Blood Pressure Percentile*	Systolic Blood Pressure by Percentile of Height, mm Hg†							Diastolic Blood Pressure by Percentile of Height, mm Hg†						
		5%	10%	25%	50%	75%	90%	95%	5%	10%	25%	50%	75%	90%	95%
12	90th	116	116	118	119	120	121	122	75	75	76	76	77	78	78
	95th	120	120	121	123	124	125	126	79	79	80	80	81	82	82
13	90th	118	118	119	121	122	123	124	76	76	77	78	78	79	80
	95th	121	122	123	125	126	127	128	80	80	81	82	82	83	84
14	90th	119	120	121	122	124	125	126	77	77	78	79	79	80	81
	95th	123	124	125	126	128	129	130	81	81	82	83	83	84	85
15	90th	121	121	122	124	125	126	127	78	78	79	79	80	81	82
	95th	124	125	126	128	129	130	131	82	82	83	83	84	85	86
16	90th	122	122	123	125	126	127	128	79	79	79	80	81	82	82
	95th	125	126	127	128	130	131	132	83	93	83	84	85	86	86
17	90th	122	123	124	125	126	128	128	79	79	79	80	81	82	82
	95th	126	126	127	129	130	131	132	83	83	83	84	85	86	86

*Blood pressure percentile was determined by a single reading.

†Height percentile was determined by standard growth curves.

(From Update on the 1987 Task Force Report on High Blood Pressure in Children and adolescents: working Group Report from the National High Blood Pressure Education Program. *Pediatrics* 1996;98:649–658, with permission.)

Table 27-2. 90th and 95th Percentile Blood Pressures for Girls Aged 1 to 17 Years by Height Percentile.

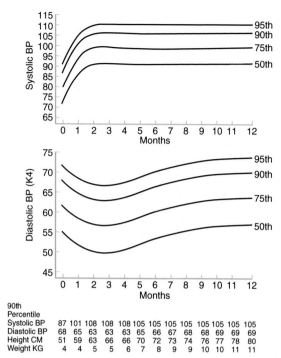

90th Percentile												
Systolic BP	87	101	108	108	108	105	105	105	105	105	105	105	105
Diastolic BP	68	65	63	63	63	65	66	67	68	68	69	69	69
Height CM	51	59	63	66	66	70	72	73	74	76	77	78	80
Weight KG	4	4	5	5	6	7	8	9	9	10	10	11	11

Figure 27-1. Age-specific percentiles of blood pressure measurements in boys—birth to 12 months of age.

(From Task Force on Blood Pressure Control in Children. Report of the second task force on blood pressure control in children—1987. *Pediatrics* 1987;79:1–25, with permission.)

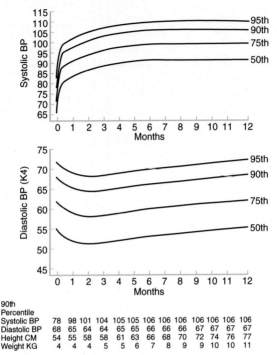

90th Percentile												
Systolic BP	78	98	101	104	105	105	106	106	106	106	106	106	106
Diastolic BP	68	65	64	64	65	65	66	66	66	67	67	67	67
Height CM	54	55	58	58	61	63	66	68	70	72	74	76	77
Weight KG	4	4	4	5	5	6	7	8	9	9	10	10	11

Figure 27-2. Age-specific percentiles of blood pressure measurements in girls—birth to 12 months of age.
(From Task Force on Blood Pressure Control in Children. Report of the second task force on blood pressure control in children—1987. *Pediatrics* 1987;79:1–25, with permission.)

References
1. Flynn JT. Evaluation and management of hypertension in childhood. *Progress Pediatr Cardiol* 2001;12:177–188.
2. Lauer RM, Clarke WR. Childhood risk factors for adult blood pressure: the Muscatine Study. *Pediatrics* 1989;84:633–641.
3. National High Blood Pressure Education Program. Update on the 1987 Task Force Report on High Blood Pressure in Children and Adolescents: a working group report from the National High Blood Pressure Education Program. National High Blood Pressure Education Program Working Group on Hypertension Control in Children and Adolescents. *Pediatrics* 1996;98:649–658.
4. Task Force on Blood Pressure Control in Children. Report of the Second Task Force on Blood Pressure Control in Children—1987. *Pediatrics* 1987;79:1–25.
5. The Fourth Report on the Diagnosis, Evaluation, and Treatment of Hypertension in Children and Adolescents. *Pediatrics* 2004;114(2):555–576.

Timothy J. Horita

Although numerous conditions can lead to overproduction of thyroid hormone (hyperthyroidism), it is fairly uncommon in the pediatric population. Most cases are due to autoimmune pathology. In the neonate born to a mother with hyperthyroidism, signs and symptoms may be noticed before birth or several days into life. Graves' disease accounts for most pediatric cases, along with toxic (uninodular or multinodular) goiter and inflammatory conditions such as thyroiditis.

Although a goiter is usually present, it may be difficult to detect on a screening examination. Other signs and symptoms of hyperthyroidism are usually quite evident. Thyroid hormone, with its many physiologic actions, often produces a state similar to sympathetic overstimulation. In noncongenital cases, symptoms are most commonly detected in the early teens, and much more commonly in girls.

The initial work-up for a child with suspected hyperthyroidism is fairly straightforward. Referral to a pediatric endocrinologist is often very helpful in co-management.

Medications Associated with Hyperthyroidism

- Dessicated thyroid extract (factitious hyperthyroidism)
- Levothyroxine sodium (factitious hyperthyroidism)
- Liothyronine sodium (factitious hyperthyroidism)
- Liotrix (factitious hyperthyroidism)
- Methimazole (may cross placenta)
- Propylthiouracil (may cross placenta)

Causes of Hyperthyroidism

- Autoimmune acute thyroiditis
- Congenital
- Factitious hyperthyroidism
- Graves' disease
- Infectious acute thyroiditis
- Iodine ingestion/toxicity
- McCune-Albright syndrome
- Pituitary resistance to thyroid hormone
- Subacute thyroiditis
- Thyroid binding globulin deficiency

- Thyroid carcinoma
- Toxic uninodular goiter (thyroid adenoma)
- Toxic multinodular goiter
- Thyroid-stimulating hormone (TSH)-secreting pituitary tumor

Key Historical Features

Symptoms of Hyperthyroidism
- Anxiety
- Irritability
- Excessive nervousness
- Excessive sweating
- Palpitations
- Increased appetite
- Weight loss or inadequate weight gain
- Decreased fat stores (newborn)
- Generalized weakness
- Generalized fatigue
- Dyspnea on exertion
- Diarrhea
- Menstrual irregularities
- Sleep difficulties
- Heat intolerance
- Eye dryness, redness, or irritation

Medical History
- Intrauterine growth retardation
- Developmental delay
- Syncope

Medications

Family History of Autoimmune Disease or Thyroid Disease

Key Physical Findings

✓ Vital signs (for elevated basal temperature, elevated heart rate, hypertension, or hypotension)

✓ General assessment for an ill or toxic appearance

✓ Thyroid examination for a goiter or lobular thyroid, thyroid tenderness, or a palpable thyroid nodule (painless or painful)

✓ Head and neck examination for exophthalmos, lid lag or lid retraction, or cervical lymphadenopathy. Also note microcephaly or evidence of craniosynostosis.

✓ Hair examination for alopecia

✓ Cardiac examination for tachycardia, murmurs, or atrial fibrillation

✓ Chest examination for gynecomastia

✓ Abdominal examination for hepatomegaly or splenomegaly

✓ Skin examination for jaundice, flushing, warmth, or excessive sweating

✓ Nail examination for thinning or splitting

✓ Neurologic examination for tremor, tongue fasciculations, hyperreflexia, clonus, or muscle weakness

Suggested Work-Up

TSH	To make the diagnosis of hyperthyroidism
Free thyroxine (T_4)	Increased in Graves' disease
Tri-iodothyronine (T_3)	Increased in Graves' disease

Additional Work-Up

Thyroid receptor antibodies (thyrotropin receptor-stimulating antibody)	Present in more than 90% of adolescents with Graves' disease but is not necessary for the diagnosis of Graves' disease
Thyroperoxidase antibody	Present in Graves' disease and chronic lymphocytic thyroiditis
Complete blood count (CBC)	Leukocytosis may occur as a result of hyperthyroidism
Calcium	If hypercalcemia is suspected as a result of hyperthyroidism
Alkaline phosphatase	May be elevated as a result of hyperthyroidism
Alanine aminotransferase (ALT), aspartate aminotransferase (AST)	Elevated liver enzymes may occur as a result of hyperthyroidism

Blood glucose	Hyperglycemia may occur as a result of hyperthyroidism
Radioactive iodine uptake scanning (or technetium-99m) scanning	Typically used when one or more thyroid nodules are palpated. Not routinely necessary in adolescents with classic features of Graves' disease
Thyroid ultrasonography	May be useful in diagnosing thyrotoxicosis by identifying nodules and goiter that may not be readily apparent on examination
Echocardiogram	If signs or symptoms of congestive heart failure are present
Plain films for bone age	Very young children with Graves' disease often have advanced skeletal maturation and craniosynostosis
Magnetic resonance imaging (MRI) of ocular muscles	If Graves' ophthalmopathy is suspected

References

1. Antoniazzi F, et al. Graves' ophthalmopathy evolution studied by MRI during childhood and adolescence. *J Pediatr* 2004;144(4):527–531.
2. Dabon-Almirante CL. Clinical and laboratory diagnosis of thyrotoxicosis. *Endocrinol Metab Clin North Am* 1998;27(1):25–35.
3. Hanna CE, LaFranchi SH. Adolescent thyroid disorders. *Adolesc Med* 2002;13(1):13–35.
4. Manji N, et al. Influences of age, gender, smoking, and family history on autoimmune thyroid disease phenotype. *J Clin Endocrinol Metab* 2006;91(12):4873–4880.
5. Nayak B, Hodak SP. Hyperthyroidism. *Endocrinol Metab Clin North Am* 2007;36:617-656.
6. Palma Sisto PA. Endocrine disorders in the neonate. *Pediatr Clin North Am* 2004;51:1141–1168.
7. Reid JR, Wheeler SF. Hyperthyroidism: diagnosis and treatment. *Am Fam Physician* 2005;72:623–630.
8. Trivalle C, et al. Differences in the signs and symptoms of hyperthyroidism in older and younger patients. *J Am Geriatr Soc* 1996;44:50–53.
9. Zimmerman D, Lteif AN. Thyrotoxicosis in children. *Endocrinol Metab Clin* 1998;27:109–126.

Timothy J. Horita

Most children begin walking unassisted between the ages of 12 and 36 months. There is wide variation within this age range and how an individual child progresses. Strength, balance, vision, coordination, and anticipation are only a few of the skills to be mastered for normal gait to be achieved. Shorter steps and a wider shifting of weight from side to side are considered normal compared with that of adults. However, certain patterns of gait abnormalities can provide critical information in detecting common pathology.

Gait is divided into **swing** and **stance** phases. The most common form of limp, an antalgic gait, is caused by pain. The time in stance phase is shortened in the painful limb, with a resulting increase in the swing phase. An acute limp implies an underlying pathology that causes disruption of the usual gait pattern.

The older patient may be able to localize a painful joint or area of pain, but referred pain patterns must also be considered. The clinician must consider the spine, pelvis, and lower extremities for a possible cause in a child with a limp. A helpful clinical "pearl" to remember is that knee pain in a child is hip pathology until proven otherwise. Because hip pathology may manifest as knee or thigh pain, the hip must always be considered in patients with knee or thigh pain. The very young child rarely is able to verbalize the location of the pain. If a previously ambulatory child prefers to crawl on his or her knees, foot pathology is more likely.

The differential diagnosis in an acutely limping child can be divided into broad categories of causes, such as traumatic, infectious, inflammatory, neoplastic, congenital, neuromuscular, and developmental. Pain that is worse in the morning suggests a rheumatologic process. Pain at night that awakens a child from sleep is worrisome for a malignant process. If a child has multiple fractures or a fracture of a suspicious nature, child abuse should be considered.

A diagnosis of **growing pains** must meet three criteria: (1) the leg pain is bilateral; (2) the pain occurs only at night; and (3) the patient has no limp, pain, or symptoms during the day.

A delay in diagnosis can be devastating in some processes, particularly a septic joint. A septic process may result in damage to the cartilaginous surface of a joint. A septic hip may result in avascular necrosis of the femoral head.

Medications Associated with Abnormal Gait

- Aminoglycosides
- Chemotherapy (many)
- Loop diuretics
- Nonsteroidal anti-inflammatory agents (NSAIDs)

- Phenytoin and other anti-siezure medications
- Quinine
- Sedatives and hypnotics
- Thalidomide

Causes of Abnormal Gait

Congenital Problems and Bone Disorders

- Clubfoot
- Congenitally short femur
- Developmental dysplasia of the hip
- Genu valgum
- Leg-length discrepancy
- Osteogenesis imperfecta
- Sickle cell disease
- Spondylolisthesis
- Tibial or femoral anteversion

Developmental

- Legg-Calvé-Perthes disease
- Osteochondritis dessicans
- Slipped capital femoral epiphysis
- Tarsal coalitions

Hematologic

- Hemophilia with hemarthrosis
- Sickle cell disease

Infection

- Cellulitis
- Diskitis
- Epidural abscess
- Gonorrhea
- Lyme disease
- Myositis
- Osteomyelitis
- Postinfectious reactive arthritis
- Rheumatic fever
- Septic arthritis
- Toxic synovitis
- Tuberculosis of bone

Inflammatory

- Henoch-Schönlein purpura
- Inflammatory bowel disease
- Juvenile rheumatoid arthritis
- Serum sickness
- Systemic lupus erythematosus
- Transient synovitis

Muscular disease

- Muscular dystrophies (many types)

Neurologic or Neuromuscular

- Agyroposis
- Ataxia-telangiectasia
- Cerebral palsy
- Flaccid paralysis
- Hereditary sensory motor neuropathies
- Herniated disc
- Hypotonia
- Spasticity
- Spinal muscular atrophy
- Tethered cord

Tumor

- Benign bone tumors
  - o Osteoblastoma
  - o Osteoid osteoma
- Malignant bone tumors
  - o Ewing's sarcoma
  - o Leukemia
  - o Lymphoma
  - o Osteosarcoma
- Spinal cord tumors

Trauma and Overuse

- Ankle sprain
- Chondromalacia patella
- Fracture
- Ligamentous injury
- Muscle hematoma

- Osgood-Schlatter disease
- Osteochondritis dessicans
- Soft tissue contusion
- Stress fracture
- Toddler's fracture

Other

- Hysteria/conversion
- Mimicry

Key Historical Features

✓ Time of onset of limp or abnormal gait

✓ Duration of the limp

✓ Getting better, getting worse, or staying the same

✓ Time of day when the pain occurs

✓ Recent trauma

✓ Painful versus painless limping

✓ Fever or chills

✓ Unexplained weight loss or lack of appropriate growth

✓ Recent viral illness

✓ Past trauma to the lower extremity or back

✓ Myalgias

✓ Morning stiffness or pain

✓ Back pain

✓ Nocturnal pain

✓ Missing school or change in normal activity

✓ Tinnitus or vertigo

✓ Symptoms better with rest or worse with strenuous activity

✓ Relative increase or decrease in physical activity

✓ Clumsiness or lack of coordination

✓ Past medical history

- Seizures
- Inflammatory or infectious disease
- Recurrent fractures or dislocations

✓ Family history of connective tissue disease

✓ Review of systems, especially fever, weight loss, rash, and gastrointestinal (GI) symptoms

Key Physical Findings

✓ Observation of gait and stance

✓ Symmetry of in-toeing, out-toeing, or toe walking

✓ Complete palpation of leg musculature for focal tenderness

✓ Examination of each joint in the legs for swelling, erythema, warmth, or tenderness

✓ Palpation of the spine for local tenderness

✓ Observation of the spine in forward flexion to evaluate range of motion and identify asymmetric turning of the spine

✓ Evaluation of spinal extension

✓ Full range of motion at the hips, knees, and ankles

✓ Measurement of thigh and calf circumference to evaluate for atrophy

✓ FABER test (hip *f*lexion, *ab*duction, and external *r*otation) to evaluate for pain in the sacroiliac joint

✓ Inspection of forefoot angle and foot shape (Figures 29-1 and 29-2)

✓ Examination of the feet for clawing of the toes or cavus foot deformity

✓ Examination of foot angle with respect to the thigh (Figure 29-3)

✓ Focused neurologic examination
  • Walking on the toes
  • Walking on the heels
  • Hopping on one foot
  • Deep tendon reflexes
  • Sensory exam

✓ Evaluation for symmetry of internal rotation of the hips by placing the child in the prone position with the knees flexed and the ankles falling away from the body (Figure 29-4)

✓ Galeazzi test to evaluate for developmental dysplasia of the hip or a leg-length discrepancy (Figure 29-5)

Initial Work-Up

Complete blood count (CBC), erythrocyte sedimentation rate (ESR), and/or C-reactive protein (CRP)	If infection or leukemia is being considered
Aspiration of the joint with fluid analysis for cell counts, Gram stain, aerobic and anaerobic cultures, protein, and glucose. Include a culture for gonorrhea if the patient is sexually active	If a septic process is suspected
Plain films of the areas in question. Films of the entire extremity should be considered for referred pain. Films of the entire extremity should be strongly considered in the nonverbal patient (a fracture is identified in 20% of these patients with a limp)	To evaluate the bones and joints

Additional Work-Up

Ultrasonography of the hip to identify fluid in the hip joint	Useful when infection of the hip is suspected
Alkaline phosphatase, calcium, electrolytes	If a neoplastic process is suspected
Serum rheumatoid factor	If inflammatory disease is suspected, though inflammatory diseases in children often are seronegative
Creatine kinase	If Duchenne muscular dystrophy is suspected
Bone scan	May be considered when the cause of a child's limp cannot be localized by history or physical examination
Computed tomography (CT) scan (best to evaluate bone structure) or magnetic resonance imaging (MRI; best to evaluate tissue)	To further evaluate bright areas on bone scan, to further evaluate a particular part of a limb in question, or to evaluate the lumbosacral spine

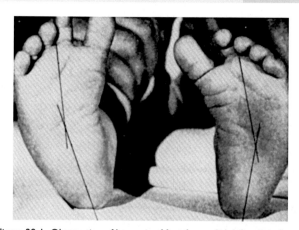

Figure 29-1. Observation of long axis of foot for medial deformity of metatarsals in relation to long axis of feet.
(From Behrman RE, Kliegman RM, Jenson HB. *Nelson Textbook of Pediatrics*, 17th ed. Philadelphia: WB Saunders; 2004:23–66.)

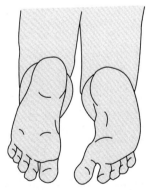

Figure 29-2. Foot shape. Using the same position for measurement of the thigh-foot angle, in Figure 29-3, the shape of the foot can also be evaluated. In this illustration, the left foot has normal alignment, whereas the right foot demonstrates metatarus adductus.
(From Behrman RE, Kliegman RM, Jenson HB. *Nelson Textbook of Pediatrics*, 17th ed. Philadelphia: WB Saunders; 2004:23–66.)

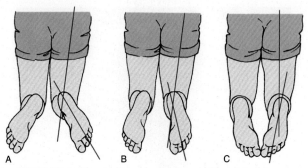

Figure 29-3. With patient in the prone position and knees flexed at 90 degrees, foot angle is observed in relation to thighs.
(From Behrman RE, Kliegman RM, Jenson HB. *Nelson Textbook of Pediatrics*, 17th ed. Philadelphia: WB Saunders; 2004:23–66.)

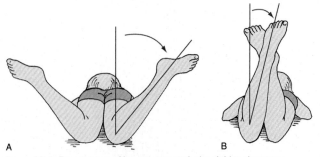

Figure 29-4. Examination of hip rotation with the child in the prone position and knees bent at 90 degrees.
(From Behrman RE, Kliegman RM, Jenson HB. *Nelson Textbook of Pediatrics*, 17th ed. Philadelphia: WB Saunders; 2004:23–66.)

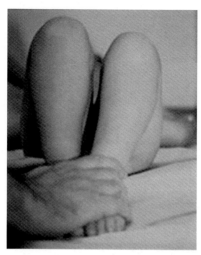

Figure 29-5. Galeazzi test.
(From Leet AI, Skaggs DL. Evaluation of the acutely limping child. *Am Fam Physician* 2000;61:1011–1018, with permission.)

References

1. Behrman RE, Kliegman RM, Jenson HB. *Nelson Textbook of Pediatrics*, 17th ed. Philadelphia: WB Saunders; 2004:23–66.
2. Casselbrant ML, Mandel EM. Balance disorders in children. *Neurologic Clin* 2005;23:807-829.
3. Crawford AH, Gabriel KR. Foot and ankle problems. *Orthop Clin North Am* 1987;18:649–666.
4. Kogan M, Smith J. Simplified approach to toe-walking. *J Pediatr Orthop* 2001;21:790-791.
5. Leet AI, Skaggs DL. Evaluation of the acutely limping child. *Am Fam Physician* 2000;61:1011–1018.
6. Thompson GH. Gait disturbances. In: Kliegman RM, ed. *Practical Strategies in Pediatric Diagnosis and Therapy*, 2nd ed. Philadelphia: WB Saunders; 2003:823–843.

Theodore X. O'Connell

Lymph nodes in children may be palpated as early as the neonatal period, and they continue to enlarge through puberty. Most normal children have palpable cervical, inguinal, and axillary adenopathy. As a general rule, a lymph node is considered enlarged if it measures more than 10 mm in its longest diameter. Exceptions to this rule include epitrochlear nodes, which are abnormal if greater than 5 mm in diameter, and inguinal nodes, which are abnormal only if greater than 15 mm in diameter. Palpable supraclavicular, iliac, and popliteal nodes should always be considered abnormal.

Hyperplastic lymph nodes that develop in response to viral infection are small, discrete, mobile, nontender, and bilateral. *Pyogenic nodes* tend to be unilateral, large, warm, and tender with surrounding erythema and edema. Chronic infections are associated with nodes with discrete margins adherent to underlying tissue and minimal signs of inflammation. Nodes associated with malignancy are generally firm, discrete, and nontender. These nodes are usually rubbery and do not have surrounding inflammation. These nodes become matted together over time and fixed to the skin or underlying structures.

In general, rapidly growing lymph nodes without a confirmed, compatible diagnosis require prompt tissue biopsy. Regressing or fluctuating lymphadenopathy usually can be observed as it is rarely associated with malignancy or serious systemic illness. However, if the lymphadenopathy persists and a diagnosis is required, biopsy is the most definitive option. Persistent lymphadenopathy beyond 8 weeks without an obvious source also should be considered for biopsy.

Causes of Lymphadenopathy

Bacterial

- Actinomycetes
- Anaerobic bacteria
- Atypical mycobacteria
- *Bartonella henselae*
- Brucellosis
- Diphtheria
- *Francisella tularensis*
- Gram-negative enterics
- Group A *streptococcus*
- *Mycobacterium tuberculosis*
- *Staphylococcus aureus*

- *Salmonella* spp.
- Syphilis
- *Yersinia* spp.

Congenital

- Branchial cleft cyst
- Bronchogenic cyst
- Cystic hygroma
- Epidermoid cyst
- Sternocleidomastoid tumor
- Thyroglossal duct cyst

Fungal

- Aspergillosis
- Blastomycosis
- Candida
- Coccidioidomycosis
- Cryptococcus
- Histoplasmosis
- Sporotrichosis

Malignancy

- Hodgkin's disease
- Leukemia
- Lymphoproliferative disorders
- Metastatic disease
- Nasopharyngeal carcinoma
- Neuroblastoma
- Non-Hodgkin's lymphoma
- Parotid tumors
- Rhabdomyosarcoma
- Thyroid tumors
- Wilms' tumor

Parasitic

- Toxoplasmosis

Viral

- Adenovirus
- Coxsackie virus

- Cytomegalovirus (CMV)
- Epstein-Barr virus
- Herpes simplex virus
- Human herpes virus 6
- Human immunodeficiency virus (HIV)
- Measles
- Mumps
- Rubella
- Varicella

Other

- Allergic diathesis
- Castleman disease
- Collagen vascular disease
- Histiocytic necrotizing lymphadenitis (Kikuchi lymphadenitis)
- Histiocytosis X
- Immunodeficiency diseases
- Kawasaki syndrome
- Reticuloendotheliosis
- Sarcoidosis
- Serum sickness
- Sinus histiocytosis with massive lymphadenopathy
- Storage disorders

Key Historical Features

✓ Onset and duration of symptoms

✓ Rate of lymph node enlargement

✓ Exposure to animal bites or scratches

✓ Weight loss

✓ Fever

✓ Malaise or fatigue

✓ Rashes

✓ Recent sore throat, cough, or upper respiratory symptoms

✓ Recent antibiotic usage (including how the symptoms and lymphadenopathy responded)

✓ Tuberculin skin test status

✓   Hemoptysis

✓   Chest pain

✓   Dysphagia

✓   Past medical history

✓   Past surgical history

✓   Family history

✓   Social history

- •   Animal exposure
- •   Risk factors for HIV infection
- •   Contact with tuberculosis
- •   Recent travel

Keys Physical Findings

✓   Vital signs

✓   General assessment of well-being

✓   Assessment of the quantity, character, and size of the enlarged nodes

✓   Thorough lymph node examination for other lymphadenopathy

✓   Evaluation of local soft tissue and skin drained by the enlarged nodes for any evidence of inflammation

✓   Evaluation of distal areas for nodule or papule formation

✓   Abdominal examination for hepatosplenomegaly

✓   Skin examination for rashes, bites, or scratches

✓   Breast examination for teenagers and college-age women if axillary lymphadenopathy is present

✓   Testicular examination if inguinal lymphadenopathy is present

Suggested Work-Up

Complete blood count (CBC)	To evaluate for infection or malignancy
Biopsy by fine-needle, core-needle, or open biopsy	If malignancy is suspected or if the diagnosis remains in doubt after a thorough evaluation

Gram stain and cultures for aerobic, anaerobic, acid-fast (tuberculous), and fungal microorganisms	After drainage when suppurative adenopathy is present
Histologic examination	If there is any suspicion of malignancy, a portion of the suppurated lymph node that is not necrotic should be examined histologically
Surgical excision with histologic examination	If atypical mycobacterial lymphadenitis is suspected
Chest radiograph and intradermal skin testing	If tuberculous lymphadenopathy is suspected
Indirect fluorescent antibody test for *Bartonella* spp. antigen	If cat scratch disease is suspected
Computed tomography (CT) scan	To evaluate large mediastinal masses
Magnetic resonance imaging (MRI)	May be a better diagnostic tool for posterior mediastinal masses
Biopsy by mediastinoscopy, thoracoscopy, or thoracotomy	If mediastinal mass/lymphadenopathy is present
Open or laparoscopic biopsy	If abdominal lymphadenopathy is present

References

1. Kelly CS, Kelly RE. Lymphadenopathy in children. *Pediatr Clin North Am* 1998;45:875–888.
2. Grossman M, Shiramizu B. Evaluation of lymphadenopathy in children. *Curr Opin Pediatr* 1994;6:68–76.

Theodore X. O'Connell

Musculoskeletal pain during childhood can be difficult for children to characterize. Most causes of acute musculoskeletal pain in children are easy to identify, but the cause of chronic musculoskeletal pain or pain that has associated systemic symptoms can be more difficult to diagnose (see Figure 31-1). Nonrheumatic causes of musculoskeletal pain are much more common than rheumatic causes.

The initial step in obtaining a history is to determine the specific location of the pain. The joint distribution and the number of joints involved should be determined. It should be determined whether the pain is localized to soft tissues rather than the joint. The possibility of referred pain should be considered.

The next step is to determine whether the cause of musculoskeletal pain may be an inflammatory process. Constitutional symptoms (fevers, fatigue, or rash), joint swelling, and prolonged morning stiffness suggest an inflammatory process. A limitation in the child's daily activities is of greater concern for an inflammatory process or malignancy. Rapid onset of pain suggests trauma, sepsis, hemarthrosis, or malignancy. Onset of pain over several days suggests an infectious or reactive arthritis.

A complete history and physical examination should be performed to help evaluate for extra-articular signs of infection, rheumatic disease, or malignancy. Laboratory tests and radiologic studies may help to support a diagnosis in a child with a high likelihood of an inflammatory process and may exclude worrisome diagnoses such as infection and malignancy. Laboratory tests and radiologic studies should be used judiciously as many have a low pretest probability in the primary care setting.

Many rheumatic processes tend to develop over weeks or months. As such, close follow-up and re-examination is helpful to determine the child's clinical course. Resolution of symptoms and absence of worrisome features are reassuring. Additional signs and symptoms present at a follow-up visit may direct additional evaluation or referrals.

Causes of Musculoskeletal Pain

Arthritides of inflammatory bowel disease

Benign hypermobility syndrome

Benign nocturnal limb pains of childhood (growing pains)

Compartment syndrome

Deep vein thrombosis

Ehlers-Danlos syndrome

Hemarthrosis

Hemophilia

Henoch-Schönlein purpura

Hernia

Infectious causes

- Acute rheumatic fever
- Brodie abscess
- Cellulitis
- Diskitis
- Gas gangrene
- Lyme disease
- Necrotizing fasciitis
- Orchitis
- Osteochondritis (Pseudomonas)
- Osteomyelitis
- Pyomyositis
- Transient synovitis

Legg-Calvé-Perthes disease

Malignancy

- Acute lymphoblastic leukemia
- Ewing's sarcoma
- Lymphoma
- Osteosarcoma
- Rhabdomyosarcoma

Marfan syndrome

Myofascial pain

Osteochondrosis

Osteomyelitis (focal and chronic recurrent multifocal)

Osteonecrosis

Patellofemoral pain syndrome

Rheumatic causes

- Ankylosing spondylitis
- Arthritis with enthesitis
- Dermatomyositis
- Juvenile dermatomyositis
- Juvenile rheumatoid arthritis (RA; pauciarticular and polyarticular)
- Mixed connective tissue disease
- Psoriatic arthritis

- Reactive arthritis (Reiter syndrome)
- Septic arthritis
- Seronegative spondyloarthropathies
- Sjögren's syndrome
- Systemic lupus erythematosus (SLE)
- Wegener's granulomatosis

Sickle cell disease

Slipped capital femoral epiphysis

Spondylolisthesis

Spondylolysis

Stress fracture

Testicular torsion

Thrombophlebitis

Trauma

- Fractures
- Sprains
- Strains

Key Historical Features

✓ Location of the pain

✓ Number of joints involved

✓ Onset of pain

✓ Frequency and duration of pain

✓ Joint distribution

✓ Number of joints involved

✓ Morning stiffness

✓ Swelling

✓ Alleviating and aggravating factors

✓ Effect on daily activities

✓ Antecedent trauma

✓ Recent illness

✓ Constitutional symptoms

- Fever
- Weight loss
- Fatigue

- ✓ Extra-articular symptoms
  - Rashes
  - Upper respiratory tract infection
  - Genitourinary infection
  - Gastrointestinal (GI) tract infection
  - Ophthalmologic symptoms such as red eye
- ✓ Past medical history
- ✓ Immunization history
- ✓ Family history
- ✓ Recent travel
- ✓ Animal exposure
- ✓ Review of systems

Key Physical Findings

- ✓ Vital signs and evaluation of growth curve
- ✓ General appearance
- ✓ Cardiac examination for murmurs
- ✓ Evaluation for lymphadenopathy
- ✓ Abdominal examination for hepatosplenomegaly
- ✓ Skin examination for rash
- ✓ Joint examination
  - Warmth
  - Swelling
  - Range of motion (ROM)
  - Guarding
  - Tenderness to palpation
  - Synovial thickening
  - Symmetry (unilateral or bilateral)
  - Skin changes overlying joints
- ✓ Musculoskeletal examination
  - Muscle atrophy
  - Muscle mass and strength
  - Bony enlargement
  - Focal tenderness or abnormalities of bones or muscles

Suggested Work-Up

Laboratory studies are used primarily for screening when the differential diagnosis includes infectious, inflammatory, or neoplastic processes. Laboratory tests and radiologic studies should be used judiciously as many have a low pretest probability in the primary care setting.

Complete blood count (CBC)	To evaluate for leukocytosis (infection, leukemia, or inflammatory conditions). White blood cell count may be normal in up to 66% of children with leukemia in the initial evaluation of chronic joint pain
Erythrocyte sedimentation rate (ESR) or C-reactive protein	To evaluate for inflammation or infection. May be normal or elevated with arthritis. A discordant ESR and platelet count is worrisome for malignancy
Antinuclear antibodies (ANA)	To evaluate for SLE, juvenile RA, and vasculitis. May be positive in up to 40% of healthy children. Titers greater than 1:320 are more likely to represent inflammatory diseases
Rheumatoid factor	To evaluate for juvenile RA. 70% sensitivity and 82% specificity for RA, but has low positive predictive value in the primary care setting
Plain radiographs	May be helpful in diagnosing fractures, bone tumors, and chronic osteomyelitis
Blood culture	If an infectious etiology is suspected
Joint aspiration and examination of the synovial fluid (cell count and differential, gram stain, glucose, protein, aerobic and anaerobic cultures)	For a child with monoarthritis, who should be considered to have septic arthritis until it is ruled out

Additional Work-Up

Lactate dehydrogenase	May be helpful when malignancy is suspected as elevated levels may indicate malignancy
Antistreptolysin-O (ASO) titer	If a recent streptococcal infection is suspected as the cause of arthritis
Lyme antibody titer	If Lyme disease is suspected
Anti-double-stranded DNA	To evaluate for SLE
HLA-B27 genotype	May be useful in the diagnosis of spondyloarthropathy. Should be considered if there is a family history of inflammatory bowel disease, psoriasis, or spondyloarthropathy
cANCA (antineutrophil cytoplasmic antibody)	To confirm a diagnosis of Wegener granulomatosis
Urinalysis and creatinine	If Henoch-Schönlein purpura is suspected
Synovial biopsy	May be necessary for the child with chronic monoarticular joint pain in whom a definitive diagnosis cannot be made after a thorough evaluation
Computed tomography (CT) scan or magnetic resonance imaging (MRI)	May be helpful in diagnosing malignancy, inflammatory conditions, and cartilage abnormalities
Technetium bone scan	May be helpful in differentiating septic arthritis from osteomyelitis. May also be useful when the source of the patient's pain is not clear after the clinical examination and initial evaluation
Ultrasonography	May be useful in identifying and quantifying a joint effusion, especially in deeper joints such as the hips. Also may be used to guide needle aspiration of these joints
Echocardiography	If pericarditis or carditis is suspected

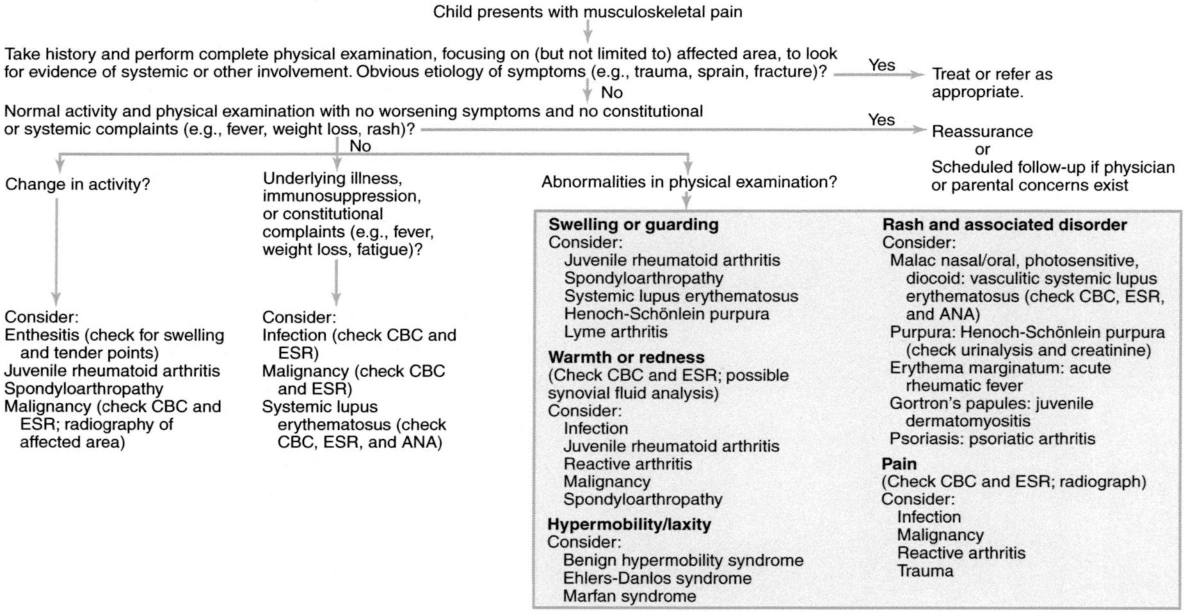

Child presents with musculoskeletal pain

Take history and perform complete physical examination, focusing on (but not limited to) affected area, to look for evidence of systemic or other involvement. Obvious etiology of symptoms (e.g., trauma, sprain, fracture)? — Yes → Treat or refer as appropriate.

No

Normal activity and physical examination with no worsening symptoms and no constitutional or systemic complaints (e.g., fever, weight loss, rash)? — Yes → Reassurance or Scheduled follow-up if physician or parental concerns exist

No

Change in activity?

Consider:
Enthesitis (check for swelling and tender points)
Juvenile rheumatoid arthritis
Spondyloarthropathy
Malignancy (check CBC and ESR; radiography of affected area)

Underlying illness, immunosuppression, or constitutional complaints (e.g., fever, weight loss, fatigue)?

Consider:
Infection (check CBC and ESR)
Malignancy (check CBC and ESR)
Systemic lupus erythematosus (check CBC, ESR, and ANA)

Abnormalities in physical examination?

Swelling or guarding
Consider:
Juvenile rheumatoid arthritis
Spondyloarthropathy
Systemic lupus erythematosus
Henoch-Schönlein purpura
Lyme arthritis

Warmth or redness
(Check CBC and ESR; possible synovial fluid analysis)
Consider:
Infection
Juvenile rheumatoid arthritis
Reactive arthritis
Malignancy
Spondyloarthropathy

Hypermobility/laxity
Consider:
Benign hypermobility syndrome
Ehlers-Danlos syndrome
Marfan syndrome

Rash and associated disorder
Consider:
Malac nasal/oral, photosensitive, discoid: vasculitic systemic lupus erythematosus (check CBC, ESR, and ANA)
Purpura: Henoch-Schönlein purpura (check urinalysis and creatinine)
Erythema marginatum: acute rheumatic fever
Gortron's papules: juvenile dermatomyositis
Psoriasis: psoriatic arthritis

Pain
(Check CBC and ESR; radiograph)
Consider:
Infection
Malignancy
Reactive arthritis
Trauma

Figure 31-1. Evaluation and diagnosis of the child with musculoskeletal pain.

References

1. Babyn P, Doria AS. Radiologic investigation of rheumatic diseases. *Pediatr Clin North Am* 2005;52:373–411.
2. Frank G, Mahoney HM, Eppes SC. Musculoskeletal infections in children. *Pediatr Clin North Am* 2005;52:1083–1106.
3. Frick SL. Evaluation of the child who has hip pain. *Orthop Clin North Am* 2006;37:133–140.
4. Gutierrez K. Bone and joint infections in children. *Pediatr Clin North Am* 2005;52:779–794.
5. Junnila JL, Cartwright VW. Chronic musculoskeletal pain in children Part I: initial evaluation. *Am Fam Physician* 2006;74:115–122.
6. Junnila JL, Cartwright VW. Chronic musculoskeletal pain in children Part II: rheumatic causes. *Am Fam Physician* 2006;74:115–122.
7. Ravelli A, Martini A. Juvenile idiopathic arthritis. *Lancet* 2007;369:767–778.
8. Tuten HR, Gabos PG, Kumar SJ, Harter GD. The limping child: a manifestation of acute leukemia. *J Pediatr Orthop* 1998;18:625–629.

Kevin Haggerty

Pediatric neck lesions may be divided into three categories: congenital, inflammatory or infectious, and neoplastic. Although most adult neck masses are malignant, 90% of pediatric neck lesions are benign. Given the diverse nature and etiologies of these lesions, no definitive or algorithmic approaches to neck masses have been established. Physicians must recognize that most of these lesions are benign and use a careful history and physical examination to guide their approach. The rapidity of onset, associated symptoms, family and social history, age of the patient, and physical findings are essential in the formulation of a differential diagnosis.

Palpable cervical nodes are present in 40% of infants. When all age groups are considered, about 55% of children have palpable nodes that are not associated with infection or systemic illness. Lymphoid tissue proliferates until puberty, at which time lymphoid mass is double that of adult values. Lymph nodes smaller than 3 mm in diameter are normal. Cervical nodes up to 1 cm in diameter are normal in children younger than 12 years of age. Small nodes in the anterior cervical triangle are usually benign.

The presence of a painless mass present at birth or identified shortly after birth is consistent with a lesion of congenital origin. Rapid enlargement often occurs with malignant lesions, inflammatory masses, and congenital masses such as thyroglossal duct cysts, branchial cleft cysts, and lymphangiomas. Acute or subacute enlargement, tenderness, and overlying erythema or fluctuance of the cervical lymph nodes, especially if temporally related to a recent upper respiratory tract infection, suggest an inflammatory origin. Cystic lesions are usually pharyngeal cleft remnants and vascular malformations, whereas solid lesions are generally inflammatory or neoplastic. Systemic symptoms may suggest a malignant or infectious process. Malignant lesions tend to be painless, solid, and associated with other systemic manifestations. Malignancy should be considered in any patient with a solitary posterior cervical mass. Supraclavicular masses are most likely to represent lymphoma.

Inflammatory or Infectious Lesions

Most pediatric cervical lymphadenopathy is not associated with systemic illness or infection. Viral upper respiratory tract infection is the most common cause of bilateral lymphadenopathy. Suppurative lymph nodes are unilateral, tender, warm nodes caused by pyogenic infection of the tonsils and pharynx.

Mycobacterial lymphadenitis is seen in children 1 to 5 years of age and is usually accompanied by symptoms consistent with a disseminated mycobacterial infection.

Bartonella henselae infection, or cat-scratch fever, most commonly presents as tender regional (usually axillary, preauricular, or cervical) lymphadenopathy 5 to 60 days after contact with affected cats. It is usually accompanied by fever, malaise, and fatigue.

Congenital Masses

Congenital masses may be present from birth or become more prominent with growth and development. Thyroglossal duct cysts are the most common congenital masses, developing between 2 and 10 years of age. They arise from the remnants of embryonic thyroid tissue and are usually located midline to left of midline, inferior to the hyoid bone. Cystic hygromas or lymphangiomas are present from birth or arise in early infancy. These lesions are soft and mobile and are usually located in the posterior triangle of the neck. Cystic hygromas arise from lymphatic tissue that did not connect to the venous system. These lesions may enlarge rapidly and cause respiratory compromise.

Neoplastic Lesions

About 5% of pediatric malignancies occur in the head and neck. Most of these lesions are lymphomas (non-Hodgkin and Hodgkin). Non-Hodgkin lymphoma most commonly is found in children under the age of 6 years, whereas Hodgkin lymphoma is more common in adolescents and teens. Both these malignancies may present as a firm, painless, unilateral, supraclavicular mass. Neuroblastoma, while the most common solid tumor in children, is not commonly found in the head and neck. Primary neuroblastoma of the neck may arise from the cervical sympathetic chain.

The head and neck are common sites for rhabdomyosarcoma. This tumor arises most commonly in children 7 to 13 years of age and often presents as a painless, firm, nonmobile enlarging neck mass.

Medications Associated with Lymph Node Enlargement

- Allopurinol
- Hydralazine
- Phenytoin

Causes of Neck Masses

Congenital Causes

- Branchial cleft cyst
- Bronchogenic cyst
- Dermoid cyst
- Hemangioma

- Laryngocele
- Lymphangioma
- Teratoma
- Thymic cyst
- Thyroglosal duct cyst

Inflammatory and Infectious Causes

- Actinomycosis
- Cat-scratch disease
- Histoplasmosis
- Ludwig angina
- *Mycobacterium tuberculosis*
- Nontuberculosis mycobacterial infections
- Reactive lymphadenopathy
- Retropharyngeal abscess
- Sarcoidosis
- Sialadenitis
- Toxoplasmosis
- Tuberculosis

Neoplastic Causes

Malignant

- Fibrosarcoma
- Hodgkin's lymphoma
- Malignant thyroid tumors
- Neuroblastoma
- Non-Hodgkin's lymphoma
- Rhabdomyosarcoma
- Thyroid cancer

Nonmalignant

- Fibroma
- Goiter
- Lipoblastoma
- Lipoma
- Paraganglioma
- Salivary gland tumor
- Thyroid goiter

Other conditions
- Hematoma
- Medications
- Subcutaneous emphysema

Key Historical Features

✓ Location of the lesion

✓ Growth pattern of the lesion

✓ Age at presentation

✓ Fever

✓ Irritability

✓ Fatigue

✓ Night sweats

✓ Weight loss

✓ Anorexia

✓ Travel

✓ Animal exposures

✓ Past medical history

✓ Past surgical history

✓ Medications

✓ Family history

✓ Social history

Key Physical Findings

✓ Vital signs

✓ Quantification of the size of the lesion

✓ Location or anatomical site of the lesion (posterior triangle, supraclavicular)

✓ Mobility or fixation to internal structures

✓ Consistency of the lesion

✓ Tenderness

✓ Surrounding skin findings and color

✓ Regional lymphadenopathy

✓ General physical examination

Table 32-1 characterizes key examination findings of common lesions.

Diagnosis	Location	Physical Findings
Branchial cleft cyst	Anterior to middle third of sternocleidomastoid muscle	Mass that may retract with swallowing. Fistula may or may not be present
Cat-scratch disease	Anterior triangle, submandibular, or preauricular	Tender lymphadenopathy
Cystic hygroma (lymphangioma)	Anterior triangle, submandibular, or preauricular	Soft spongy mass, nontender. May increase in size with Valsalva maneuver. Can be differentiated from hemangioma in that it transilluminates
Dermoid cyst	Midline lesions	Mobile, painless, firm mass. Does not move with tongue protrusion
Hemangioma	May occur at various locations on neck and face	Soft mobile mass that increases in size with Valsalva maneuver. Red/bluish. Does not transilluminate
Lymphadenitis	Multiple inflamed masses in the anterior and posterior triangle	Painful, erythematous, fluctuant nodes. Patient may have fever; may drain purulent fluid
Lymphoma	Occipital and supraclavicular	Large, firm, usually painless mass
Mycobacterial and granulomatous infections	Cervical, submandibular, supraclavicular	Painful, may be erythematous, may have draining sinus tract
Rhabdomyosarcoma	Parameningeal sites (posterior aspect of neck), multiple locations	Painless, rapidly enlarging mass
Thyroglossal duct cyst	Anterior neck, submental and midline	Firm mass that retracts with tongue protrusion

Table 32-1. Key Examination Findings of Common Lesions

Suggested Work-Up

The history and physical examination may provide adequate information to assess the risk of serious disease. Children with presumed bacterial lymphadenitis or a low-risk mass of undetermined causation without significant findings may be placed on a trial of antibiotics and observation. This trial should not exceed 2 weeks.

Complete blood count (CBC)	If an infection or malignant process is suspected
Purified protein derivative (PPD) tuberculin test	If mycobacterial infection is suspected. The test will be negative in 50% of cases of atypical mycobacterial infection
Erythrocyte sedimentation rate (ESR), C-reactive protein	May be useful in characterizing the neck mass as part of a systemic illness

Chest radiograph	If malignancy or mycobacterial infection is suspected
Ultrasonography	To distinguish between a cystic lesion and a solid mass. Helpful in differentiating congenital cystic masses from solid lymph nodes and neoplasms
Fine needle aspiration or open biopsy	May be required to establish the diagnosis, especially when other diagnostic tests are unrevealing and the mass persists or increases in size. See Table 32-2

Additional Work-Up

Serologic studies	If toxoplasmosis, histoplasmosis, cytomegalovirus infection, or Epstein-Barr virus infection is suspected
Bartonella henselae antibody	If cat-scratch disease is suspected
Wound cultures	Useful in cases of suppurative lymphadenitis to identify a pathogen and choose an appropriate antibiotic
Rheumatoid factor and antinuclear antibodies	If a rheumatologic process is suspected
Computed tomography (CT) scan	More effective than ultrasonography in identifying deeper, less well-defined lesions
Magnetic resonance imaging (MRI) of neck masses	Becoming more widely used early in the evaluation
Thyroid scan and/or thyroid function tests	If thyroglossal duct cyst is suspected
Sialography	If sialadenitis is suspected
Arteriography	May be helpful in evaluating hemangioma

1. Palpable node is present in a neonate.
2. Node has increased in size after 2 weeks.
3. Node has not decreased in size after 4 to 6 weeks.
4. After 8 to 12 weeks, node has not regressed to a size that is believed to be within normal limits for the child's age and the site of involvement.
5. Signs of serious disease are present that indicate the need for early biopsy.
   a. Progressively enlarging firm to hard node greater than 2 cm in diameter.
   b. Supraclavicular adenopathy in the absence of pulmonary infection.
   c. Persistent fever or weight loss.
   d. Fixation of the node to adjacent tissue.
   e. Node located in the posterior triangle or in some atypical site, such as deep to the sternomastoid muscle or in the middle portion of the back.

*When other diagnostic tests are unrevealing, biopsy may be required to rule out malignancy and establish the diagnosis.

Table 32-2. Criteria for Cervical Lymph Node Biopsy*

References

1. Brown RL, Azizkhan RG. Pediatric head and neck lesions. *Pediatr Clin North Am* 1998;45:889–905.
2. Jordan N, Tyrell J. Management of enlarged cervical lymph nodes. *Curr Paediatr* 2004;14:154–159.
3. Kelly CS, Kelly RE. Lymphadenopathy in children. *Pediatr Clin North Am* 1998;45:875–888.
4. Park YW. Evaluation of neck masses in children. *Am Fam Physician* 1995;51:1904–1911.
5. Zitelli BJ. Evaluating the child with a neck mass. *Contemp Pediatr* 1990;7:90–112.

33 NOCTURNAL ENURESIS

Jonathan M. Wong

Enuresis refers to the persistence of inappropriate voiding of urine beyond the age of anticipated bladder control, which is age 4 to 5 years at the latest. The International Children's Continence Society, in order to standardize the diagnosis, has defined *nocturnal enuresis* as "the involuntary loss of urine that occurs only at night. It is normal voiding that happens at an inappropriate and socially unacceptable time and place." In the past, various classification schemes were also used to describe this problem such as nocturnal versus diurnal, primary versus secondary, and uncomplicated versus complicated.

Children are not considered to be enuretic until they have reached 5 years of age. Mentally disabled children should have reached a mental age of four years before being considered enuretic. A child of 5 to 6 years of age has nocturnal enuresis if he or she has two or more bedwetting episodes per month. A child older than 6 years of age has nocturnal enuresis if he or she has one or more wetting episodes per month.

Nocturnal enuresis affects some five to seven million children in the United States, making it the most common pediatric urologic complaint. At 5 years of age, 15% to 25% of children still wet the bed; males predominate. The spontaneous resolution rate of nocturnal enuresis is about 15% per year. Thus, 8% of 12-year-old boys and 4% of 12-year-old girls are enuretic. Only 1% to 3% of adolescents are still wetting the bed.

Despite its prevalence, nocturnal enuresis is not completely understood, and the condition is believed to be multifactorial. Organic causes are responsible for nocturnal enuresis in fewer than 5% of cases. Such organic causes should be searched for and ruled out if the history suggests their presence.

Medications Associated with Nocturnal Enuresis

Diuretics

Causes of Nocturnal Enuresis

The current belief is that enuresis is a multifactorial condition involving genetic, familial, psychological, urologic, and hormonal factors. It is also likely related to a maturational delay in affected patients. The following is a list of causes:

Alcohol

Caffeine

Chronic constipation

Diabetes insipidus

Diabetes mellitus

Ectopic ureter

Familial causes

Foods that increase nocturnal urine production

- Chocolate
- Citrus juices
- Dairy products

Genetic causes

- Positive family history in 65%-85% of bedwetting patients

Hormonal causes

- It is postulated that normal development includes the establishment of a circadian rhythm in the release of arginine vasopressin, the antidiuretic hormone. Patients with nocturnal enuresis may be delayed in achieving this circadian rise, and hence develop nocturnal polyuria.

Irregular food and drink intake

Neurogenic bladder

Posterior urethral valves

Psychological causes

- Although nocturnal enuresis was once thought to be the result of psychological problems, it is now believed that these problems are the result of bedwetting.
- Bedwetting is not thought to be an act of rebellion.

Sleep arousal dysfunction

Urinary tract infection (UTI)

Urologic causes

- Diminished functional bladder capacity

Key Historical Features

The history and physical examination should be directed at excluding causes of complicated enuresis, such as spinal cord injuries (neurogenic bladder), UTI, posterior urethral valves in boys, and ectopic ureter in girls. A voiding diary may be helpful in quantifying the historical information.

✓ Detailed toilet training history

✓ Onset and pattern of wetting

✓ Number of dry nights per month

✓ Most consecutive dry nights

- ✓ Evening fluid intake
- ✓ Bladder emptied at bedtime
- ✓ Voiding behavior, especially small frequent voids that suggest bladder instability or small functional bladder capacity
- ✓ Urine stream
- ✓ Sleep pattern
- ✓ Parasomnias
- ✓ Daytime urinary symptoms
- ✓ Dysuria
- ✓ Bowel habits, especially constipation
- ✓ Encopresis
- ✓ Family's and patient's attitude toward the bedwetting
- ✓ Polyuria/number of times per day that the child voids
- ✓ Polydipsia
- ✓ Gait disturbance
- ✓ Nighttime snoring
- ✓ Present and past treatments for nocturnal enuresis and their results
- ✓ Medical history
  - Neurologic problems
  - Injury to the genital or back area
- ✓ Birth history, especially any complications
- ✓ Surgical history
- ✓ Family medical history
- ✓ Social history

Key Physical Findings

- ✓ Head and neck examination for evidence of mouth breathing
- ✓ Abdominal and flank examination for the presence of masses, including an enlarged bladder or constipation
- ✓ Examination of the lower back for evidence of spinal dysraphism
- ✓ Urogenital examination for evidence of abuse or any physical abnormalities
- ✓ Gait evaluation for evidence of neurologic deficits
- ✓ Extremity evaluation of muscle tone and strength

✓   Reflexes (including cremasteric, anal, abdominal, and deep tendon) to evaluate the functioning of the spinal cord in the pelvic region

✓   Rectal examination if the history suggests encopresis or constipation

Suggested Work-Up

Urinalysis	To assess specific gravity (for diabetes insipidus) and urinary glucose level (for diabetes mellitus) as well as to evaluate for the presence of infection or blood

If the history, physical examination, and urinalysis do not suggest a secondary cause of nocturnal enuresis, no further work-up is needed.

Additional Work-Up

Urine culture	If symptoms suggest a UTI or if the urinalysis suggests infection
Voiding cystourethrogram and renal ultrasound	To evaluate for vesicoureteral reflux if the urine culture reveals an infection
Serum glucose	If the history or urinalysis suggests diabetes mellitus
Sleep study	If a sleep disorder is suspected

References

1. Lawless MR, McElderry DH. Nocturnal enuresis: current concepts. *Pediatr Rev* 2001;22: 399–407.
2. Schmitt BD. Nocturnal enuresis. *Pediatr Rev* 1997;18:183–191.
3. Thiedke CC. Nocturnal enuresis. *Am Fam Physician* 2003;67:1499–1506.

Jonathan M. Wong

Pediatric obesity is defined as a weight that is 20% or more above the mean weight for children of the same height. *Severe obesity* is defined as a weight that is 40% above the mean weight for children of the same height. Alternatively, a weight greater than the 85th percentile or the 95th percentile may be used to define obesity and severe obesity, respectively. However, this latter definition does not differentiate lean body mass from fat.

The prevalence of childhood obesity has risen significantly in the United States over the past several decades. According to the National Health Examination Survey Cycles, the prevalence of pediatric obesity is estimated to be 25% to 30%. This represents an increase of 54% in children aged 6 to 11 and 39% in adolescents 12 to 17 years old. From 1976 to 2000, the prevalence of severe obesity increased even more, with Hispanic, Native American, and black patients preferentially affected.

The persistence of obesity into adulthood depends on several factors, including the age at which the child becomes obese, the severity of the obesity, and the prevalence of obesity in at least one parent. A child with one obese parent is three times more likely to become obese, whereas a child with two obese parents is 10 times more likely to become obese. Interestingly, children younger than 3 years who are overweight do not have a higher incidence of future obesity unless one parent is obese. After age 3, the likelihood that obesity will persist into adulthood increases with advancing age of the child (50% in a child age 6, and 70% to 80% in adolescents).

Several studies suggest that obese children, on average, do not consume significantly more calories than their nonobese peers. However, a modest increase in calories consumed over time equates to the increase in weight seen in these patients. An increase of 50 to 100 calories per day can result in a 5- to 10-pound weight gain over the course of 1 year.

Evaluation of obesity in childhood is important for preventing disease progression with its associated morbidities into adulthood. These morbidities include hypertension, type 2 diabetes mellitus, hyperlipidemia, hyperuricemia, and some forms of cancer. Obesity may also have a negative impact on self-esteem of children and adolescents.

Although genetic and hormonal causes of obesity are rare, they do warrant consideration in obese children. It is important to differentiate between endogenous and idiopathic causes of obesity. Endogenous causes represent fewer than 10% of all cases of pediatric obesity. With endogenous causes, the child is typically of short stature (less than the 10th percentile), often is mentally impaired, may have delayed bone age, and there is no family history of obesity. In idiopathic cases, the child usually has normal stature, a family history of obesity, normal mental function, normal or advanced bone age, and a normal physical examination.

Medications Associated with Childhood Obesity

- Antipsychotic agents
- Corticosteroids
- Cyproheptadine
- Methimazole
- Progestins
- Propylthiouracil
- Valproate

Causes of Childhood Obesity

Only a small percentage of cases of childhood obesity are associated with a hormonal or genetic defect, with the rest being environmental or idiopathic in nature.

Hormonal Causes

- Acquired hypothalamic problems (brain injury, brain tumor, cranial irradiation)
- Cushing's disease
- Hypothyroidism
- Primary hyperinsulinism
- Pseudohypoparathyroidism

Genetic Causes

- Alstrom syndrome
- Beckwith-Wiedemann syndrome
- Börjeson-Forssman-Lehmann syndrome
- Cohen syndrome
- Familial lipodystrophy
- Laurence-Moon/Badet-Biedl syndrome
- Prader-Willi syndrome
- Ruvalcaba syndrome
- Sotos' syndrome
- Turner's syndrome
- Weaver syndrome

Key Historical Features

✓ Nutritional history
- Breastfeeding or formula
- Duration of breastfeeding

- Age at introduction of solids
- Caloric intake
- Dietary quality in terms of nutrient balance and food groups

✓ Level of physical activity

✓ Limitations because of weight

✓ Amount of sedentary activity such as watching television or playing video games

✓ Respiratory difficulties such as snoring and somnolence

✓ Perinatal history
- Birth weight
- Maternal gestational diabetes

✓ Past medical history
- Diabetes
- Asthma or breathing difficulties

✓ Psychiatric history
- Depression
- Self-esteem
- Eating disorders

✓ Menstrual history in females

✓ Medications

✓ Family history
- Obesity
- Diabetes
- Cardiovascular disease

✓ Social history
- Living situation
- Socioeconomic status
- Who prepares the food
- Frequency of dining out or eating fast food
- Tobacco use
- Alcohol use

Key Physical Findings

✓ Vital signs, including blood pressure

✓ Height and weight

✓   Evaluation of the growth curve

✓   May consider triceps skin fold

✓   General evaluation to assess for any dysmorphisms

✓   Head and neck examination for tonsillar hypertrophy or thyroid goiter

✓   Pulmonary examination for evidence of asthma, decreased air exchange, or hypoventilation syndromes

✓   Abdominal examination to evaluate for central versus peripheral obesity or right upper quadrant tenderness suggesting the presence of gallstones

✓   Musculoskeletal examination to assess for stress on the joints, especially the knees

✓   Genitourinary examination to evaluate for hypogonadism

✓   Neurologic examination to evaluate mental status and evidence of any genetic syndromes

✓   Skin examination for acne, acanthosis nigricans, fungal infections, or striae

✓   Vision and hearing screening if a genetic syndrome is suspected

Suggested Work-Up

If the history or physical examination suggests an endogenous cause for obesity, the work-up should be guided by clinical suspicion.

Fasting blood sugar	May be indicated in obese children because the rates of juvenile-onset type 2 diabetes mellitus are rising
Fasting lipid panel	The National Cholesterol Education Program Expert Panel on Blood Cholesterol Levels in Children and Adolescents recommended screening in all obese children over 2 years of age
Thyroid-stimulating hormone (TSH) and free thyroxine (T_4)	To evaluate for hypothyroidism
Dexamethasone suppression test and 24-hour free urinary cortisol level	If Cushing's disease is suspected

Fasting blood sugar, plasma insulin, and C-peptide levels	If hyperinsulinism is suspected
Calcium, phosphorous, and parathyroid hormone (PTH) levels	If pseudohypoparathyroidism is suspected
Brain imaging	If a hypothalamic cause is suspected
Genetic testing/chromosomal analysis (genetic syndromes)	If a genetic syndrome is suspected

Additional Work-Up

Follicle-stimulating hormone (FSH) and luteinizing hormone (LH)	If polycystic ovary syndrome is suspected
Sleep study	If sleep apnea is suspected
Pulmonary function tests	If asthma is suspected
Liver function tests	If nonalcoholic fatty liver disease is suspected
Right upper quadrant ultrasound	If cholelithiasis is suspected

References

1. Barlow SE, Dietz WH. Obesity evaluation and treatment: expert committee recommendations. *Pediatrics* 1998;102:E29.
2. Moran R. Evaluation and treatment of childhood obesity. *Am Fam Physician* 1999;59: 861–868.
3. Policy Statement by Committee on Nutrition. Prevention of pediatric overweight and obesity. *Pediatrics* 2003;112:424–430.
4. Speiser PW, et al. Consensus statement: childhood obesity. *J Clin Endocrinol Metab* 205;90:1871–1887.

Theodore X. O'Connell

Normal puberty begins between 8 and 14 years of age in girls and between 9 and 14 years of age in boys. Girls begin puberty with breast buds and skeletal growth, followed by the arrival of pubic hair, axillary hair, and menarche. Boys have testicular enlargement followed by the appearance of pubic hair, enlargement of the penis, and spermarche. The age at which pubertal milestones are attained varies among the population studied. In addition, it is influenced by activity level and nutritional status. Girls with low body fat may have a significant delay in menarche (up to a year or longer), whereas obese girls may have earlier onset of puberty.

Precocious puberty is defined as the development of secondary sexual characteristics before the age of 8 years in girls and 9 years in boys. It involves not only early physical changes of puberty, but also linear growth acceleration and acceleration of bone maturation, which leads to early epiphyseal fusion and short adult height.

There are two types of precocious puberty. *Central precocious puberty* (gonadotropin-releasing hormone [GnRH]-dependent precocious puberty) results from premature activation of the hypothalamic GnRH pulse generator-pituitary gonadotropin-gonadal axis. In *peripheral precocious puberty*, (GnRH-independent precocious puberty), sex steroid secretion is independent of the GnRH pulse generator. Pathologic causes of puberty are likely if sexual development occurs in very young children or if there is contrasexual development. Peripheral causes are always pathologic and tend to produce an atypical puberty with loss of synchronicity of pubertal milestones.

Central precocious puberty is more common by far in girls than in boys, and in girls it is idiopathic 95% of the time. Boys more commonly (i.e., more than 50%) have an identifiable pathologic peripheral cause for precocious puberty. Therefore, all boys with precocious puberty should undergo detailed investigation. In girls, additional investigation can be based on the clinical impression. Central nervous system (CNS) disorders account for a higher percentage of cases in boys but must also be excluded in girls.

Pubertal variants cause isolated development of one of the secondary sexual characteristics without accelerated skeletal maturation. Occasionally they can progress to precocious puberty.

Simple premature thelarche involves only breast development (unilateral or bilateral), without pubic hair growth, without accelerated bone maturation, and with a normal height outcome. No treatment is required. The disorder is usually self-limited and can resolve spontaneously or persist to normal puberty.

Simple premature adrenarche involves only pubic or axillary hair development, without the other manifestations of puberty. No treatment is required, although late-onset congenital adrenal hyperplasia should be ruled out with a measurement of the serum 17α-hydroxyprogesterone level. There is an increased incidence of simple premature adrenarche in patients with CNS abnormalities.

Unilateral or bilateral gynecomastia may occur in boys as puberty begins. In fact, this is a nearly universal finding among boys in middle to late puberty. It usually resolves within 2 years. Pathologic gynecomastia occurs in Klinefelter's syndrome, prolactin-secreting adenomata, and as a result of drugs such as marijuana and phenothiazines.

Patients with precocious puberty and pubertal variants require an initial bone age as a baseline. In precocious puberty, the bone age is usually accelerated more than two standard deviations above the chronological age. In pubertal variants, the bone age should be within two standard deviations of the chronological age. The bone age should be obtained at periodic intervals to determine whether pubertal variants have progressed to precocious puberty. The bone age is also used to monitor the effectiveness of therapy. Additional evaluation of precocious puberty is outlined below.

Medications Associated with Precocious Puberty

Androgens

Estrogens

Causes of Precocious Puberty (Adapted from Tables 1 and 2 in Fahmy)

GnRH-Dependent Precocious Puberty

CNS tumors

- Astrocytoma
- Craniopharyngioma
- Ependymoma
- Hamartoma of the tuber cinereum
- Hypothalamic and optic gliomas
- Pinealoma

Previous CNS injury

- Cranial radiation
- Head trauma
- Hypoxic-ischemic encephalopathy
- Infections (abscess, encephalitis, meningitis)

Other CNS disorders

- Arachnoid cyst
- Developmental abnormalities
- Hydrocephalus

- Neurofibromatosis type I
- Sarcoid granuloma
- Septo-optic dysplasia
- Tuberculous granuloma
- Tuberous sclerosis

GnRH-Independent Precocious Puberty

Females

- Autonomously functioning ovarian cysts
- Feminizing adrenal tumor
- Ovarian tumors
  - o Carcinoma
  - o Cystadenoma
  - o Gonadoblastoma
  - o Granulosa-theca cell tumors
- Peutz-Jeghers syndrome

Males

- Gonadotropin-secreting tumors
  - o CNS tumors
    - Chorioepithelioma
    - Germinoma
    - Teratoma
  - o Tumors outside the CNS
    - Choriocarcinomas
    - Hepatoblastoma
    - Hepatoma
    - Teratomas
- Increased androgen secretion by adrenal or testes
  - o Congenital adrenal hyperplasia (21- or 11ß-hydroxylase deficiency)
  - o Familial testotoxicosis
  - o Leydig cell tumor
  - o Virilizing adrenal tumor

Both sexes

- Hypothyroidism
- Iatrogenic or exogenous sexual precocity
- McCune-Albright syndrome
- Severe hypothyroidism

Key Historical Features

✓ Previous growth and development

✓ Sequence of pubertal events

✓ Past medical history

✓ Past surgical history

✓ Medications

✓ Detailed dietary history in underweight or overweight children

✓ Family history, especially of genetic disease or precocious or delayed puberty

Key Physical Findings

✓ Vital signs

✓ Evaluation of growth chart

✓ Head and neck examination to evaluate the optic fundi, estimate the visual fields, and evaluate the sense of smell

✓ Determination of the Tanner stage of pubertal development

✓ Breast examination for pubertal development and asymmetry

✓ Genital examination for pubertal development and testicular abnormalities

Suggested Work-Up

Radiograph of the left wrist	To estimate physiologic age for comparison with the child's chronologic age
Serum follicle-stimulating hormone (FSH) and luteinizing hormone (LH), estradiol, testosterone, thyroid-stimulating hormone (TSH), thyroxine (T_4), and human chorionic gonadotropin (hCG)	To confirm the impression of idiopathic precocious puberty, to localize the abnormality of the pathologic cause of precocious puberty, or to guide the choice of imaging study
Serum 17-hydroxyprogesterone and dehydroepiandrosterone (DHEA)	If a peripheral cause is suspected or if virilization is present in a female patient

Pelvic ultrasound

Used to determine whether pubertal changes have occurred in the uterus and ovaries. Also indicated if a peripheral cause (ovarian tumor) is suspected

Additional Work-Up

Magnetic resonance imaging (MRI) of the brain and pituitary gland

If a central pathologic cause is suspected on the basis of hormone measurements. Also indicated in boys with elevated hCG levels

GnRH stimulation test

100 µg of GnRH is administered either intravenously or subcutaneously after an overnight fast. Serum levels of FSH and LH are measured at baseline just before the injection and at 15, 30, 45, and 60 minutes after the injection. Test interpretation is controversial, but a twofold to threefold rise in FSH and LH may be observed if the patient has central precocious puberty. A peak LH level of more than 15 international units per liter or a peak LH-to-peak FSH ratio of more than 0.66 are also criteria for defining a pubertal GnRH test

Breast ultrasound

Indicated in unilateral or asymmetric premature thelarche to exclude masses

Testicular ultrasound

Indicated if asymmetric enlargement of the testes is present

Skeletal survey or radionuclide bone scan

Indicated for patients with McCune-Albright syndrome to evaluate for lesions of fibrous dysplasia

References

1. Bates GW. Hirsutism and androgen excess in childhood and adolescence. *Pediatr Clin North Am* 1981;28:513–530.
2. Blondell RD, Foster MB, Dave KC. Disorders of puberty. *Am Fam Physician* 1999;60: 209–224.
3. Fahmy JL, Kaminsky CK, Kaufman F, Nelson MD, Parisi MT. The radiological approach to precocious puberty. *Br J Radiol* 2000;73:560–567.
4. Klein KO. Precocious puberty: who has it? who should be treated? *J Clin Endocrinol Metab* 1999;84:411–414.

Theodore X. O'Connell

Most healthy children excrete small amounts of protein in the urine, which is called *physiologic proteinuria*. Physiologic proteinuria varies with age and the size of the child. When corrected for body surface area, the protein excretion is highest in newborn infants and decreases with age until late adolescence, when adult levels are reached. *Asymptomatic or isolated proteinuria* is defined as proteinuria not associated with any signs or symptoms of renal disease. The estimated prevalence of isolated asymptomatic proteinuria in children is between 0.6% and 6.3%. However, only 0.1% of children have persistent proteinuria.

In general, the finding of proteinuria does not warrant an extensive work-up. The finding of proteinuria must be confirmed on two or three more occasions. *Transient proteinuria,* the most common cause in children, can be induced by a variety of factors, including fever and exercise. The finding of at least two positive urine tests out of three specimens suggests persistent proteinuria and warrants additional evaluation. Orthostatic proteinuria occurs when urine protein excretion occurs in the upright position but returns to normal when the patient is recumbent.

The diagnostic evaluation of the child with dipstick-positive proteinuria is affected by the presence or absence of symptoms. Isolated asymptomatic proteinuria on a urine dipstick, without hematuria, hypertension, or signs of systemic illness or stress, is detected in about 15% of adolescent patients. Only about a fourth of patients have a second dipstick positive for protein if reevaluated within 48 hours, and an even smaller percentage remain positive if tested serially over 6 to 12 months. Therefore, the first step in the evaluation of a child or adolescent with isolated proteinuria is to determine whether the patient has persistent proteinuria in at least two of three urine samples tested 1 or more weeks apart.

Once the diagnosis of persistent proteinuria is established, the physician should determine whether the patient has *orthostatic (postural) proteinuria.* Orthostatic proteinuria accounts for about 60% of children with persistent proteinuria. The patient is instructed to empty the bladder at bedtime, and in the morning a urine sample is immediately collected, which is then tested for protein. Another urine sample is obtained later in the day after ambulation. If the morning urine samples are negative or show trace protein while ambulatory ones are 1+ or greater, a diagnosis of orthostatic proteinuria is made, and no further evaluation is required. However, a urine protein-creatinine ratio should be measured and blood pressure obtained yearly for children diagnosed with orthostatic proteinuria.

If the patient has persistent, nonorthostatic proteinuria, a more thorough evaluation is warranted. This includes quantification of proteinuria using either a 24-hour urine collection or a urine protein-creatinine ratio on a spot sample. The urine protein-creatinine ratio has become the preferred method because it is more reliable than 24-hour urinary protein measurements. In adults and children over 2 years of age, a urine protein-creatinine ratio lower than 0.2 on a random urine specimen obtained during the day is considered normal. In children aged 6 to 24 months, the upper limit of normal is 0.5. A ratio above 3.0 is consistent with nephrotic-range proteinuria.

The symptomatic child requires more aggressive clinical evaluation. Symptoms may be nonspecific (fever, malaise), more specific but nonurinary (arthritis, rash), or urinary specific (edema, hypertension). The underlying disorder may be renal in origin or secondary to a systemic disease. Children with heavy proteinuria and edema should be evaluated promptly for nephrotic syndrome and, if it is present, have consultation with a pediatric nephrologist. Children with non–nephrotic-range persistent proteinuria who present with hypertension, an abnormal urinalysis, or an elevated plasma creatinine concentration should be evaluated by a pediatric nephrologist.

Figure 36-1 provides an algorithm for the evaluation of pediatric proteinuria.

Causes of Proteinuria

Benign persistent proteinuria

Orthostatic (postural) proteinuria

Transient proteinuria

- Abdominal surgery
- Congestive heart failure
- Emotional stress
- Epinephrine administration
- Extreme cold exposure
- Fever
- Hypovolemia
- Seizures
- Strenuous exercise

Glomerular proteinuria

- Alport syndrome
- Congenital nephrotic syndrome
- Diabetes mellitus
- Focal segmental glomerulonephritis
- Henoch-Schönlein purpura
- Hepatitis B virus-associated nephropathy
- Human immunodeficiency virus (HIV)-associated nephropathy

- IgA nephropathy
- Lupus glomerulonephritis
- Membranoproliferative glomerulonephritis
- Membranous glomerulonephritis
- Minimal change nephrotic syndrome
- Postinfectious glomerulonephritis

Tubulointerstitial proteinuria

- Chronic interstitial nephritis
- Cystinosis
- Heavy metal poisoning
- Medications (antibiotics, antineoplastic agents)
- Obstructive uropathy
- Polycystic kidney disease
- Pyelonephritis
- Reflux nephropathy
- Renal dysplasia
- Toxins
- Wilson's disease

Key Historical Features

✓ Recent history of fever, strenuous exercise, dehydration, emotional distress, or exposure to cold

✓ Recent upper respiratory infection

✓ Gross hematuria

✓ Change in weight

✓ Change in urine output

✓ Symptoms of a systemic illness

- Fevers
- Arthralgias
- Arthritis
- Skin rash

✓ Hearing loss

✓ Medical history, especially recurrent urinary tract infections (UTIs)

✓ Surgical history

✓ Medications

✓ Family history, especially familial renal disease

Key Physical Findings

✓   Vital signs, especially blood pressure

✓   Measurement of height and weight

✓   General assessment of physical condition

✓   Cardiopulmonary examination

✓   Abdominal examination for ascites and to palpate the kidneys

✓   Extremity examination for edema or arthritis

✓   Skin examination for rash, purpura, or pallor

Suggested Work-Up

Repeat urine dipstick two or three additional times	To determine whether proteinuria is persistent
Perform urine dipstick on a morning urine sample and a sample later in the day	To determine whether orthostatic proteinuria is the cause

If orthostatic proteinuria is diagnosed, the child should be reevaluated annually with measurement of blood pressure and urine protein-creatinine ratio. If fixed isolated proteinuria is diagnosed, the work-up depends on the degree of proteinuria. If the urine protein-creatinine ratio is less than 1.0, twice-yearly visits, later extended to annual visits, with determination of the urine protein-creatinine ratio are sufficient. If proteinuria persists beyond 1 year, referral to a pediatric nephrologist for renal biopsy should be considered. If the urine protein-creatinine ratio is greater than 1.0, the following evaluation should be considered:

Microscopic urinalysis	To evaluate the urinary sediment for hematuria, bacteria, casts, or eosinophils
Serum blood urea nitrogen (BUN) and creatinine	To evaluate renal function
Serum electrolytes	To evaluate for electrolyte disturbances
Serum albumin and total protein	Serum albumin is decreased in nephrotic syndrome

Complete blood count (CBC)	To evaluate for infection. Anemia may indicate chronic renal disease
Serum cholesterol and triglycerides	Cholesterol is increased in nephrotic syndrome
Complement C3 and C4 levels	Levels are decreased in the glomerulonephritides
Renal ultrasound	To help detect anatomic or congenital abnormalities, especially in children under 6 years of age

Additional Work-Up

Antistreptolysin O (ASO) titer and/or streptozyme test	If postinfectious glomerulonephritis is suspected by history. Referral to a pediatric endocrinologist is recommended for most cases of postinfectious glomerulonephritis
Antinuclear antibody (ANA)	If systemic lupus erythematosus is suspected
Hepatitis B and C serologies	If hepatitis B or C infections are suspected
HIV testing	If HIV infection is suspected
Voiding cystourethrogram	May be indicated if there is a history of recurrent UTIs or if a renal ultrasound reveals scarring
Renal biopsy	May be indicated when laboratory tests are abnormal and a glomerular disease is suspected
Referral to a pediatric nephrologist	See text for some indications. Generally indicated if renal biopsy is needed, if the patient has hematuria with symptoms of renal disease, if nephrotic-range proteinuria is diagnosed, or if the diagnosis is unclear

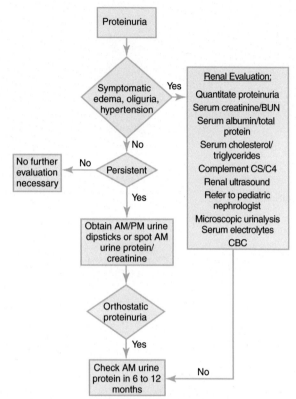

Figure 36-1. Evaluation of pediatric proteinuria.
(From Mahan JD, Turman MA, Mentser MI. Evaluation of hematuria,
proteinuria, and hypertension in adolescents. *Pediatr Clin North Am*
1997;44:1573–1589.)

References

1. Hogg RJ, et al. National Kidney Foundation's kidney disease outcomes initiative clinical
   practice guidelines for chronic kidney disease in children and adolescents: evaluation,
   classification, and stratification. *Pediatrics* 2003;111:1416–1421.
2. Hogg RJ. Adolescents with proteinuria and/or the nephrotic syndrome. *Adolesc Med Clin*
   2005;16:163–172.
3. Loghman-Adham M. Evaluating proteinuria in children. *Am Fam Physician* 1998;58:1145–1152.
4. Mahan JD, Turman MA, Mentser MI. Evaluation of hematuria, proteinuria, and hypertension
   in adolescents. *Pediatr Clin North Am* 1997;44:1573–1589.
5. Patel HP. The abnormal urinalysis. *Pediatr Clin North Am* 2006;53:325–337.

Theodore X. O'Connell

Purpura is the appearance of red or purple discolorations on the skin, resulting from the extravasation of blood from the vasculature into the skin or mucous membranes. Purpura may be classified according to their size as petechiae (less than 2 mm in diameter), purpura (2 mm to 1 cm in diameter), or ecchymoses (larger than 1 cm in diameter). Purpuric lesions do not blanch with pressure.

Purpura are not dangerous but may be the sign of a serious or life-threatening disorder. Purpura may result from a defect in platelets, plasma coagulation factors, or blood vessels. In general, petechiae and mucosal bleeding result from platelet disorders. Ecchymoses and hemarthrosis usually result from coagulation disorders. Palpable purpura result from vasculitic disorders.

Figure 37-1 provides an algorithm for the diagnosis of purpura in child.

Medications Associated with Purpura

- Alkylating agents (decreased platelet formation)
- Antimetabolites (decreased platelet formation)
- Anticonvulsants (decreased platelet formation)
- Aspirin (platelet dysfunction)
- Atropine (vascular purpura)
- Chloral hydrate (vascular purpura)
- Chlorothiazide diuretics (decreased platelet formation)
- Cimetidine (immune thrombocytopenia)
- Clofibrate (platelet dysfunction)
- Corticosteroid therapy long term (defective vascular support tissue)
- Estrogens (decreased platelet formation)
- Furosemide (platelet dysfunction)
- Heparin (immune thrombocytopenia, platelet dysfunction)
- Nitrofurantoin (platelet dysfunction)
- Nonsteroidal anti-inflammatory drugs (NSAIDs; platelet dysfunction)
- Penicillin (immune thrombocytopenia)
- Quinidine (immune thrombocytopenia)
- Sulfonamides (immune thrombocytopenia)
- Sympathetic blockers (platelet dysfunction)
- Valproic acid (immune thrombocytopenia)

Causes of Purpura

Coagulation Disorders

Acquired coagulation factor deficiency
- Circulating anticoagulants
- Disseminated intravascular coagulopathy
- Liver disease
- Uremia
- Vitamin K deficiency

Hereditary deficiency of any coagulation factor. The most common are:
- Factor VIII deficiency
- Factor IX deficiency
- von Willebrand's disease

Platelet dysfunction
- Bernard-Soulier disease
- Chronic liver disease
- Glanzmann thrombasthenia
- Storage pool disease
- Uremia

Thrombocytopenia
- Chronic idiopathic thrombocytopenic purpura
- Congenital amegakaryocytic thrombocytopenia
- Cytomegalovirus infection
- Disseminated intravascular coagulopathy
- Fanconi anemia
- Giant hemangioma (Kasabach-Merritt syndrome)
- Granulomatosis
- Hemolytic-uremic syndrome
- Herpes virus infection
- Histiocytosis
- Human immunodeficiency virus (HIV) infection
- Idiopathic (immune) thrombocytopenic purpura
- Infections (viral and bacterial)
- Leukemia
- Malignancy
- Medications
- Myelofibrosis
- Neonatal autoimmune thrombocytopenia

- Neonatal isoimmune (alloimmune) thrombocytopenia
- Neuroblastoma
- Post-transfusion purpura
- Purpura fulminans
- Splenomegaly
- Storage diseases
- Systemic lupus erythematosus
- Thrombocytopenia-absent radii syndrome
- Thrombotic thrombocytopenic purpura
- Wiskott-Aldrich syndrome

Vascular Factors

Ehlers-Danlos syndrome

Henoch-Schönlein purpura

Hereditary hemorrhagic telangiectasia

Measles

Mechanical causes

- Child abuse
- Coin rubbing
- Cupping
- Factitious purpura
- Spoon scratching
- Violent coughing or vomiting

Meningococcal infection

Psychogenic purpura

Rickettsial diseases

Scarlet fever

Typhoid

Key Historical Features

✓ Onset and duration

✓ Location of bleeding

✓ Antecedent viral infection

✓ Fever

✓ Lethargy

✓ Weight loss

✓ Bone pain

- ✓ Joint pain
- ✓ Abdominal pain
- ✓ Blood in stools
- ✓ Polyuria
- ✓ Polydipsia
- ✓ Past medical history, especially liver disease, renal disease, or lupus
- ✓ Birth history
- ✓ Maternal history if purpura has neonatal onset
- ✓ Past surgical history
- ✓ Medications
- ✓ Family history

Key Physical Findings

- ✓ Vital signs, noting fever or hypertension
- ✓ Growth parameters and comparison with previous measurements
- ✓ General evaluation of well-being
- ✓ Complete skin examination for purpura, pallor, rash, jaundice, café au lait spots, or telangiectasias
- ✓ Evaluation for lymphadenopathy
- ✓ Abdominal examination for tenderness or hepatosplenomegaly
- ✓ Genitourinary examination for scrotal edema
- ✓ Extremity examination for edema, palmar erythema, or evidence of hemarthrosis

Suggested Work-Up

Complete blood count (CBC)	To evaluate for thrombocytopenia or anemia
Peripheral blood smear	To evaluate for schistocytes suggesting hemolytic-uremic syndrome, thrombotic thrombocytopenia purpura, or disseminated intravascular coagulopathy. To evaluate for neutrophilia suggesting an infection

| Prothrombin time (PT) | To evaluate for a deficiency involving coagulation factors II, V, VII, X, or fibrinogen |

| Activated partial thromboplastin time (aPTT) | To evaluate for a deficiency involving coagulation factors II, V, VIII, IX, X, XI, XII, or fibrinogen |

Additional Work-Up

| Bleeding time | Rarely indicated in children. Measures the interval required for bleeding to stop after a standardized incision is made on the forearm |

| Measurements of specific coagulation factors or von Willebrand factor | To confirm a specific factor deficiency or von Willebrand disease |

| Platelet aggregation tests using activators, clot retraction, prothrombin consumption test, and serotonin release | If a platelet function defect is suspected |

| Bone marrow biopsy | If a second bone marrow cell line is depressed or if the cause of thrombocytopenia is not clear after initial evaluation |

| Rheumatoid factor and antinuclear antibody | If the patient has arthritis or arthralgias |

| Urinalysis | To evaluate for hematuria if Henoch-Schönlein purpura, systemic lupus erythematosus, or hemolytic-uremic syndrome is suspected |

| Blood urea nitrogen (BUN), creatinine, and urinalysis | If renal disease is suspected |

| Liver function tests | If liver disease is suspected |

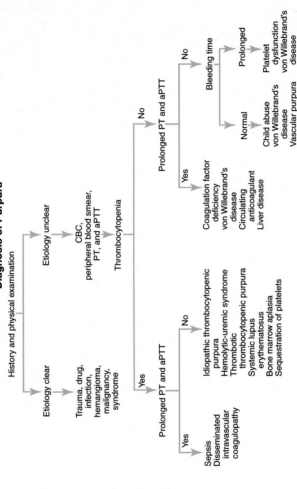

Figure 37-1. Algorithm for the diagnosis of purpura in children. PT, prothrombin time; aPTT, activated partial thromboplastin time.

Abdominal ultrasonography or computed tomography (CT) scanning	If organomegaly is present
Cranial ultrasound	To evaluate for intracranial bleeding if the neonatal platelet count is less than 50×10^3 per μL

References

1. Bolton-Maggs HB. Idiopathic thrombocytopenic purpura. *Arch Dis Child* 2000;83:220–222.
2. Cines DB, Blanchette VS. Immune thrombocytopenic purpura. *N Engl J Med* 2002;346: 995–1008.
3. Cohen AR, et al. Rash—purpura. In: Fleisher GA, Ludwig S, eds. *Textbook of Pediatric Emergency Medicine*, 3rd ed. Baltimore: Williams & Wilkins; 1993:430–438.
4. Leung AKC, Chan KW. Evaluating the child with purpura. *Am Fam Physician* 2001;64: 419–428.
5. Roberts I, Murray NA. Neonatal thrombocytopenia: causes and management. *Arch Dis Child Fetal Neonatal Ed* 2003;88:359–364.
6. Tizard J. Henoch-Schönlein purpura. *Arch Dis Child* 1999;80:380–383.

Theodore X. O'Connell

Evaluation of a scrotal mass should include classifying it as extratesticular or intratesticular, solid or cystic, and painless or painful. A painful scrotal mass requires immediate action because torsion of the spermatic cord is a urologic emergency. The dictum that a painful scrotal mass is torsion until proven otherwise should be heeded. Other painful scrotal lesions include orchitis, epididymitis, trauma, incarcerated hernia, torsion of the appendix testis or appendix epididymis, and acute bleeding into a testicular tumor.

Masses that arise from the testicle are more likely to represent malignancies, whereas extratesticular masses are more likely to be benign. An intratesticular lesion should be considered a malignancy unless proven otherwise. Solid masses are much more likely to represent neoplastic conditions, especially when painless. Transillumination using a handheld light source may help to differentiate between solid and cystic structures. Extratesticular tumors are uncommon but do occur in the form of paratesticular rhabdomyosarcoma and adenomatoid tumors of the epididymis.

Cystic lesions of the scrotum are much more common than solid lesions. A cystic mass within the epididymis is usually a spermatocele. A cyst within the spermatic cord usually represents a hydrocele. A cystic mass that surrounds the entire testicle usually represents a hydrocele. When careful physical examination, including transillumination, fails to distinguish the exact location and nature of the lesion, then scrotal ultrasonography is of great value, especially when the testis is not palpable and a hydrocele is present. Ultrasonography can confirm the location of the mass and differentiate between solid and cystic lesions.

Most extratesticular masses are benign, and most intratesticular lesions are malignant. Sonography has been shown to have nearly 100% sensitivity for detecting testicular neoplasia. Testicular microlithiasis is a rare finding that can be associated with subsequent development of germ cell tumors of the testis. Careful follow-up is warranted if testicular microlithiasis is found on ultrasonography.

The most common painless scrotal masses in infants, children, and adolescents include indirect inguinal hernias, hydroceles, varicoceles, and spermatoceles. Testicular tumors, perinatal testicular torsion, acute idiopathic scrotal edema, and soft tissue tumors of the spermatic cord are less common causes. Figure 38-1 provides a clinical approach to the painless scrotal mass.

A testicular tumor usually presents as a painless mass, although the patient may complain of scrotal heaviness or a dull ache. Physical examination should be performed with the patient in the upright and supine position because communicating hydroceles, hernias, and varicoceles

are accentuated in the upright position and with the Valsalva maneuver.
If testicular cancer is suspected, the patient should also be examined for
lymphadenopathy, gynecomastia, and abdominal masses.

Cystic and Painless Extratesticular Masses

Hernias and hydroceles represent the greatest percentage of scrotal
masses in pediatric patients. The incidence of inguinal hernias in the pediatric
population is 10 to 20 per 1000 live births. Prematurity and low birth weight
significantly increase the risk for hernias. Pediatric hernias and hydroceles are
seen as bulges or swelling in the groin or scrotum and may be more visible
when the child is crying.

A hydrocele is a collection of peritoneal fluid between the layers of the
tunica vaginalis surrounding the testicle, with or without communication
with the abdomen. A hydrocele usually presents as a painless scrotal
swelling that can be transilluminated. The presence of an inguinal hernia
or communicating hydrocele in the pediatric age group is an indication
for surgical repair because of the risk of development of incarceration or
strangulated hernia.

A varicocele is present in up to 20% of all males and is a tortuous and
dilated pampiniform venous plexus and internal spermatic vein. Varicoceles
often are described as a "bag of worms" superior to and distinct from the
testicle. Varicoceles usually first appear near midpuberty and are rarely
detected before 10 years of age. Most varicoceles occur on the left side and
usually are asymptomatic. Varicoceles have been associated with male-factor
infertility and may result in growth arrest of the left testicle. The dilatation
and tortuosity are most noticeable when the patient is upright and may
be accentuated if the patient performs a Valsalva maneuver. Once a scrotal
mass has been identified as a varicocele, it is important to assess its effects
on testicular size. A volume difference of greater than 2 cm^3 is considered
significant and serves as the minimal requirement for surgical repair of the
adolescent varicocele. If a right-sided varicocele is identified, vena cava
obstruction must be ruled out.

Spermatoceles and epididymal cysts usually present as a painless cystic
mass superior and posterior to the testis. This mass is separate from the
testis, is freely mobile, and transilluminates easily. No surgical intervention is
necessary if the spermatocele is small and painless. However, larger lesions
may cause discomfort, in which case scrotal exploration and excision may
be indicated.

Solid Painless Extratesticular Masses

The epididymis, spermatic cord, and scrotal wall may be the source of
various lesions that manifest as solid scrotal or inguinal masses. Solid lesions
of the epididymis are most commonly benign, but malignancy cannot be
excluded on clinical grounds. The adenomatoid tumor constitutes 70% of the

benign lesions. Because of the possibility of paratesticular rhabdomyosarcoma, solid extratesticular lesion must be approached surgically.

Paratesticular rhabdomyosarcoma is the most common malignant paratesticular lesion presenting as a scrotal mass in childhood. The age of incidence ranges from infancy to early adulthood. The identification of a solid extratesticular lesion is managed by radical orchiectomy. A metastatic evaluation, including computed tomography (CT) scan of the chest and retroperitoneum, is performed if the diagnosis of rhabdomyosarcoma is made. Bone marrow examination and bone scans may be indicated.

Acute idiopathic scrotal edema most commonly affects boys between 2 and 11 years of age. It is a self-limited disorder resulting in scrotal erythema and swelling that manifests as a scrotal mass. Acute idiopathic scrotal edema occurs unilaterally two thirds of the time and bilaterally in one third of cases. Examination reveals thickened, edematous scrotal skin. The testis may not be palpable; however, the testis, epididymis, and tunica vaginalis are normal. If the testis cannot be palpated, ultrasonography reveals normal testicular parenchyma and blood flow but thickened scrotal skin. Urinalysis and white blood cell count (WBC) are normal. Acute idiopathic scrotal edema usually resolves in 72 hours and always by 4 days, although recurrence may occur.

Painless Intratesticular Masses

Testicular tumors in infants and children represent only 1% of all pediatric solid tumors. The most common presentation is a painless scrotal mass. The presence of a secondary hydrocele may lead to misdiagnosis, so ultrasonography should be performed on all painless scrotal masses if the testis is not palpable because of a hydrocele.

The initial evaluation of a child with a solid testicular mass includes a thorough physical examination as outlined below. If an intratesticular mass is seen on ultrasound, α-fetoprotein (AFP) may be helpful in identifying a yolk sac carcinoma (see below), but surgery is required to establish a histologic diagnosis.

Teratoma is the second most common prepubertal testis tumor and is one of the few tumors that may be seen in the neonatal period. It is managed with radical orchiectomy or testis-sparing surgery.

Gonadal stromal tumors represent 8% of prepubertal testicular tumors and may result in signs of precocious puberty because of their hormonal activity. Leydig cell tumors often produce testosterone, whereas Sertoli cell tumors are most often hormonally inactive, though they may be associated with gynecomastia.

Gonadoblastoma is a rare tumor that occurs in patients with intersex and dysgenetic gonads.

Acute lymphoblastic leukemia with infiltration of the testis may present as a prepubertal testicular mass and should be suspected in a patient with known history of leukemia who has painless testicular enlargement.

Neonatal torsion may be the result of prenatal torsion noted at birth with a painless scrotal mass or as postnatal torsion presenting with torsion after normal scrotal testes have been documented. Neonatal torsion classically presents as a hard, nontender testicular mass noted at birth that does not transilluminate. Ultrasonography shows mixed echogenicity of the testicular parenchyma with an absence of testicular blood flow. Because the testis is almost always nonviable, exploration can be performed electively with orchiopexy of the remaining solitary testis. If the infant had a documented normal testis at birth and suffered perinatal torsion, emergency inguinal exploration is necessary.

Causes of Scrotal Masses

Painful

- Epididymitis
- Hemorrhage into tumor
- Henoch-Schönlein purpura
- Incarcerated hernia
- Kawasaki disease
- Orchitis
- Torsion of the appendix testis
- Torsion of the epididymitis
- Torsion of the spermatic cord
- Trauma (contusion, rupture, or hematoma)

Painless

- Acute idiopathic scrotal edema
- Adenomatoid tumor epididymis
- Benign soft tissue tumors
- Epidermoid cyst
- Hematocele
- Hernia
- Hydrocele
- In utero torsion
- Leiomyoma
- Lipoma
- Malignant yolk sac tumor
- Mesothelioma
- Paratesticular rhabdomyosarcoma
- Spermatocele

- Stromal tumor
- Teratoma
- Varicocele

Key Historical Features

✓ Duration of the mass

✓ Pain

✓ Constitutional symptoms such as weight loss, fever, chest pain, cough, headache

✓ Past medical history

✓ Past surgical history

✓ Family history

Key Physical Findings

✓ Careful palpation and identification of the intrascrotal contents

✓ Testicular examination for volume, masses, or tenderness

✓ Evaluation of the contralateral testis for bilateral testicular lesions

✓ Transillumination of the testicular mass

✓ Palpation of the epididymis

✓ Assessment of the spermatic cord

✓ Cremasteric reflex

✓ Examination of the inguinal canals for a hernia or cord tenderness

✓ Valsalva maneuver to evaluate for hernia or varicocele

✓ Signs of precocious puberty

✓ Abdominal examination for masses

✓ Breast examination for gynecomastia

✓ Lymph node examination, especially supraclavicular

Suggested Work-Up

Scrotal ultrasound	To help define suspected lesions and differentiate between intratesticular and extratesticular lesions

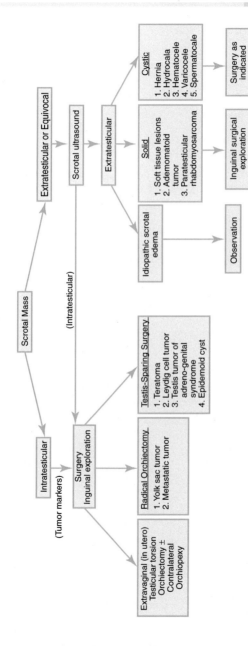

Figure 38-1. Clinical approach to the painless scrotal mass.

(From Skoog SJ. Benign and malignant pediatric scrotal masses. *Pediatr Clin North Am* 1997;44:1229–1250, with permission.)

Additional Work-Up

Serum AFP	Elevated in more than 80% of patients with yolk sac testicular tumors. It is not elevated in pediatric patients with testicular teratomas. Normal serum levels of AFP remain elevated for the first 8 months after birth
Serial follow-up and serum AFP	If testicular microlithiasis is seen in association with testicular enlargement
Chest radiography and CT scan of the abdomen and chest	Indicated if the diagnosis of a yolk sac tumor is made
Serum human chorionic gonadotropin (hCG)	Little or no value in pediatric patients

References

1. Haynes JH. Inguinal and scrotal disorders. *Surg Clin North Am* 2006;86:371–381.
2. Jayanthi VR. Adolescent urology. *Adolesc Med Clin* 2004;15:521–534.
3. Junnila J, Lassen P. Testicular masses. *Am Fam Physician* 1998;57:685–692.
4. Skoog SJ. Benign and malignant pediatric scrotal masses. *Pediatr Clin of North Am* 1997;44:1229–1250.

Timothy J. Horita and Theodore X. O'Connell

Seizures are the most common pediatric neurologic disorder, with 4% to 10% of children suffering at least one seizure in the first 16 years of life. The incidence is highest in children younger than 3 years of age and decreases with increasing age. A *seizure* is defined as a transient, involuntary alteration of consciousness, behavior, motor activity, sensation, or autonomic function caused by a paroxysmal electrical discharge of neurons in the brain. A postictal period of decreased responsiveness usually follows most seizures, and the duration of the postictal period is proportional to the duration of seizure activity. *Epilepsy* describes a condition of susceptibility to recurrent seizures. *Status epilepticus* refers to continuous or recurrent seizure activity lasting longer than 30 minutes without recovery of consciousness.

Classification systems have been developed to standardize the terminology used to describe seizure activity. Two overall seizure types exist: *partial* and *generalized.* Partial seizures originate in one cerebral hemisphere. Partial seizures are further subdivided based on whether they result in an altered level of consciousness. A *simple partial seizure* has no impairment of consciousness and most commonly manifests as abnormal motor activity. Autonomic, somatosensory, and psychic symptoms can also occur. A *complex partial seizure* occurs when an alteration of consciousness is present. An *aura* consisting of abnormal perception or hallucination often precedes this type of seizure. Both simple and complex partial seizures may ultimately become generalized.

A generalized seizure involves both cerebral hemispheres and may involve a depressed level of consciousness. Generalized seizures are either *convulsive,* with bilateral motor activity, or *nonconvulsive.* Types of generalized seizures include tonic-clonic (also known as *grand mal*), tonic, clonic, myoclonic, atonic-akinetic (drop attacks), or absence (petit mal).

The immature neonatal brain is more excitable than that of an older child and is more susceptible to seizure activity. However, the resulting seizures may be subtle and difficult to discern from other normal newborn movements or activities. Lip smacking, eye deviations, or apneic episodes may be the only manifestations of seizure activity in this age group.

A seizure represents a clinical symptom of an underlying pathologic process with many possible causes. These causes are outlined below. When a child presents with a seizure, every effort should be made to determine the cause. It is important to differentiate between a seizure and other nonepileptic conditions that may mimic seizure activity.

The topic of febrile seizures is reviewed in Chapter 17.

Medications and Toxins Associated with Seizures

Analgesics

- Meperidine
- Propoxyphene
- Salicylates
- Tramadol

Anticonvulsants (from withdrawal)

- Carbamazepine
- Phenytoin

Cellular Asphyxiants

- Azides
- Carbon monoxide
- Cyanide
- Hydrogen sulfide

Drugs of Abuse

- Amphetamines
- Cocaine
- γ-Hydroxybutyratic acid (GHB)

Envenomations

- Elapid
- Scorpion

Heavy Metals

- Arsenic
- Lead
- Thallium

Plants, Herbs, and Natural Products

- Ephedra
- *Gyromitra esculenta* mushroom
- Nicotine
- Water hemlock

Psychiatric Medications

- Buproprion
- Cyclic antidepressants

- Lithium
- Olanzapine
- Phencyclidine
- Phenothiazines
- Selective serotonin reuptake inhibitors (SSRIs)
- Venlafaxine

Rodenticides

- Bromethalin
- Zinc phosphide

Withdrawal

- Anticonvulsants
- Baclofen
- Ethanol
- Sedative-hypnotics

Miscellaneous

- Alcohol
- Anticholinergics
- Antihistamines
- Boric acid
- Camphor
- Diphenhydramine
- Fluoride
- Hypoglycemics
- Iron
- Isoniazid
- Lidocaine and local anesthetics
- Methylxanthines
  - Theophylline
  - Caffeine
- Organochlorine pesticides
  - Dichlorodiphenyltrichloroethane (DDT)
  - Lindane
- Organophosphates and carbamates
- Quinine
- Salicylates

- Sympathomimetics
- Thujone

Causes of Seizures

Infectious

- Brain abscess
- Encephalitis
- Febrile seizure
- Meningitis
- Neurocysticercosis

Neurologic, Congenital, or Developmental

- Benign neonatal convulsions
- Benign partial epilepsy of childhood
- Benign rolandic epilepsy
- Birth injury
- Cerebral palsy
- Congenital anomalies
- Degenerative cerebral disease
- Hypoxic-ischemic encephalopathy
- Infantile spasms (West's syndrome)
- Juvenile myoclonic epilepsy of Janz
- Lennox-Gastaut syndrome
- Neurocutaneous syndromes
  - Neurofibromatosis type I
  - Sturge-Weber syndrome
  - Tuberous sclerosis
- Ventriculoperitoneal shunt malfunction

Metabolic

- Hypercarbia
- Hypocalcemia
- Hypoglycemia
- Hypomagnesemia
- Hypoxia
- Inborn errors of metabolism
- Pyridoxine deficiency

Obstetric (Eclampsia)

Oncologic

Traumatic or Vascular

- Cerebral contusion
- Cerebrovascular accident
- Child abuse
- Head trauma
- Intracranial hemorrhage

Toxicologic (See Medications and Toxins Associated with Seizures)

Idiopathic (60%–70%) or Epilepsy

Differential Diagnosis of Seizures

Disorders with Altered Consciousness

- Apnea and syncope
- Breath-holding spells
- Cardiac dysrhythmias
- Migraine

Paroxysmal Movement Disorders

- Acute dystonia
- Benign myoclonus
- Pseudoseizures
- Shuddering attacks
- Spasmus mutans
- Tics

Sleep Disorders

- Narcolepsy
- Night terrors
- Sleepwalking

Psychological Disorders

- Anorexia nervosa
- Attention deficit hyperactivity disorder
- Bulimia nervosa
- Conversion disorder
- Hyperventilation

- Hysteria
- Panic attacks

Gastroesophageal Reflux (Sandifer Syndrome)

Key Historical Features

✓ Events immediately before the onset of the episode

✓ Thorough description of the seizure
- Duration
- Movements
- Loss of consciousness
- Cyanosis
- Eye findings
- Presence of an aura
- Tongue biting
- Incontinence
- Length of the postictal period
- Post-seizure neurologic abnormalities

✓ Precipitating factors
- Trauma
- Ingestions
- Fever
- Recent immunizations
- Recent illness

✓ Medications

✓ Herbal supplements

✓ Home remedies

✓ History of seizure disorder, including:
- Age of onset
- Frequency of seizures
- Whether the recent seizure was different from previous seizures
- Medications being taken for seizures
- Compliance with medication regimen
- Any recent medication changes
- Identified triggers for seizures such as sleep deprivation, flashing lights, hyperventilation

✓   Maternal exposures

✓   Birth history and perinatal complications

✓   Medical history, especially:

- Neurologic disease
- Presence of ventriculoperitoneal shunt
- Developmental delay

✓   Cognitive behavioral history, especially:

- Motor and speech milestones
- Sudden loss of speech, activity, attention
- Developmental delay

✓   Family history, especially family history of seizures

✓   Social history, especially risk for child abuse or neglect

✓   Travel history

Key Physical Findings

✓   Vital signs, including temperature, heart rate, and blood pressure

✓   Measurement of head circumference in infants

✓   Pulse oximetry

✓   General evaluation for toxic appearance or pallor

✓   Head examination for dysmorphic features, syndromic facies, signs of trauma, a bulging fontanelle, or the presence of a ventriculoperitoneal shunt

✓   Eye examination for papilledema or retinal hemorrhages

✓   Ear examination for hemotympanum

✓   Neck examination for signs of meningeal irritation

✓   Abdominal examination for hepatosplenomegaly

✓   Skin examination for petechial rash, unexplained bruising, café-au-lait spots (neurofibromatosis), adenoma sebaceum or ash leaf spots (tuberous sclerosis), or port wine stains (Sturge-Weber syndrome)

✓   Thorough neurologic examination for focal or lateralizing deficits

Suggested Work-Up of Pediatric Seizures

Laboratory testing for a child who has an afebrile seizure should be guided by the history and physical examination and should attempt to elucidate a treatable cause of seizure activity.

Bedside glucose test	To evaluate for hypoglycemia
Specific drug level(s)	Should be obtained in patients who are taking anticonvulsant medications
Electrolytes, calcium, magnesium	Indicated in patients with a history of diabetes or metabolic disorder, dehydration, excess free water intake, prolonged seizure, an altered level of consciousness, and those younger than 6 months because of an increased risk of electrolyte disturbances
Complete blood count (CBC)	If an infectious cause of the seizure is suspected
Toxicology screen	If toxin exposure is suspected
Lumbar puncture	Should be considered in patients with meningeal signs, altered mental status, a prolonged postictal period, a petechial rash, or in neonatal seizures
Brain computed tomography (CT)	Should be performed in patients with: • A history of trauma • Neurocutaneous disease • Ventriculoperitoneal shunt • Exposure to cysticercosis • Evidence of increased intracranial pressure (ICP) • Focal seizure activity • Focal neurologic deficits • Prolonged postictal period Should be considered in patients with: • Hypercoagulable states such as sickle cell disease or with oral contraceptive use • Bleeding disorder • Immunocompromised state such as human immunodeficiency virus (HIV) or malignancy

Outpatient electroencelphalography (EEG)	Indicated for children with a first-time unprovoked nonfebrile seizure

Additional Work-Up of Pediatric Seizures

Blood amino acids, lactate, pyruvate, ammonia, and urine organic acids	If an inborn error of metabolism is suspected
Emergent EEG	For patients in whom the diagnosis of nonconvulsive status epilepticus is suspected or in those with refractory seizure activity
Magnetic resonance imaging (MRI)	More sensitive than a cranial CT scan for the detection of certain tumors and vascular malformations
HIV test	If HIV infection is suspected

Suggested Work-Up of Neonatal Seizures

Serum glucose

Serum electrolytes

Serum calcium

Serum magnesium

CBC

Blood culture

Urinalysis

Urine culture

Toxicology screens

Cerebrospinal fluid cell counts, culture, and herpes simplex virus polymerase chain reaction should be considered

Blood amino acids, lactate, pyruvate, ammonia, and urine organic acids should be evaluated if an inborn error of metabolism is suspected

References

1. Blumstein MD. Childhood seizures. *Emerg Med Clin North Am* 2007;25(4):1061–1086.
2. Burkhard PR, Burkhardt K, Haenggeli CA, Landis T. Plant-induced seizures: reappearance of an old problem. *J Neurol* 1999;246:667–670.
3. Datta A, Sinclair DB. Benign epilepsy of childhood with rolandic spikes: typical and atypical variants. *Pediatr Neurol* 2007;36(3):141–145.
4. Friedman MJ, Sharieff GQ. Seizures in children. *Pediatr Clin North Am* 2006;53(2):257–277.
5. Froberg B, Ibrahim D, Furbee RB. Plant poisoning. *Emerg Med Clin North Am* 2007;25(2):375–433.
6. Wills B, Erickson T. Chemically induced seizures. *Clin Lab Med* 2006;26(1):185–209.

Timothy J. Horita

Speech and language delay affects 5% to 8% of preschool children and often persists into the school years. As a child develops from newborn to infant to toddler, there is a significant change in how the child communicates. This development continues through adulthood, but this early period is considered very important, if not critical. Numerous different areas are involved with speech and language development, and problems occur in many different ways. To communicate with others, we need to be able to produce and receive speech and language. In addition, many layers of cognitive and social development need to be mastered. *Speech* (the production of sounds) and *language* (those rules which govern communication both verbal and nonverbal) develop very early. Some of the most complex and intricate aspects of communication are not learned, or detected, until later in development.

Speech refers to the mechanics of oral communication; *language* encompasses the understanding, processing, and production of communication. Speech problems may include stuttering or dysfluency, articulation disorders, or unusual voice quality. Language problems can involve difficulty with grammar, words or vocabulary, the rules and system for speech sound production, units of word meaning, and the use of language, particularly in social contexts. Speech and language problems can exist together or separately.

Parents who have concerns about their child's development of speech and language should be taken very seriously. These concerns are usually expressed before 3 years of age. Many parents, especially those with multiple children, are able to detect these problems early on. A good familiarity with what is normal versus abnormal is very important. Several behavioral problems might be first interpreted as a speech or language disorder.

The distinction between delay versus disorder and expressive versus receptive problems is also important in the evaluation and management of children with potential problems. A *delay* is a slower than expected chronologic progression, whereas a *disorder* is a change in the actual ability to communicate in a specific area. *Expressive problems* are those involved with producing speech and language while *receptive problems* refer to the ability to receive and understand speech and language. Recognition of these problems can often provide clues to other developmental abnormalities and is important because early recognition and intervention can often be very beneficial. Although learning disorders can lead to speech and language disorders, the opposite is true as well.

A thorough developmental history is very important in making the appropriate diagnosis. Special attention should be paid to language milestones. The physician should be concerned if the child is not babbling by the age of 12 to 15 months, comprehending simple commands by 18 months of age, talking by 2 years of age, making sentences by 3 years of age, or telling a simple story by 4 to 5 years of age. Other items of concern include unintelligible speech after 3 years of age or speech that is more than a year late in comparison with normal patterns of speech development.

A basic knowledge of speech milestones is necessary to determine whether a child has speech delay. These speech milestones are presented in Table 40-1. Children's speech and language can be evaluated at any age when there is a suspicion of delay or disorder. The most common referral is to a speech-language pathologist for an evaluation. If the speech-language service does not have audiology services, a referral should be made to an audiologist or an otologist for a hearing evaluation.

Age	Achievement
1–6 mo	Coos in response to voice
6–9 mo	Babbling
10–11 mo	Imitation of sounds; says "mama/dada" without meaning
12 mo	Says "mama/dada" with meaning; often imitates two- and three-syllable words
13–15 mo	Vocabulary of four to seven words in addition to jargon; <20% of speech understood by strangers
16–18 mo	Vocabulary of 10 words; some echolalia and extensive jargon; 20% to 25% of speech understood by strangers
19–21 mo	Vocabulary of 20 words; 50% of speech understood by strangers
22–24 mo	Vocabulary >50 words; two-word phrases; dropping out of jargon; 60% to 70% of speech understood by strangers
2 to 2 1/2 yr	Vocabulary of 400 words, including names; two- to three-word phrases; use of pronouns; diminishing echolalia; 75% of speech understood by strangers
2 1/2–3 yr	Use of plurals and past tense; knows age and sex; counts three objects correctly; three to five words per sentence; 80% to 90% of speech understood by strangers
3–4 yr	Three to six words per sentence; asks questions, converses, relates experiences, tells stories; almost all speech understood by strangers
4–5 yr	Six to eight words per sentence; names four colors; counts 10 pennies correctly

Information from Schwartz ER. Speech and language disorders. In: Schwartz MW, ed. *Pediatric Primary Care: A Problem Oriented Approach.* St. Louis: Mosby; 1990:696–700.)

Table 40-1. Pattern of Speech Development

Medications Associated with Speech and Language Problems

Antibiotics

- Aminoglycosides (primarily gentamicin)
- Metronidazole

Diuretics
- Ethacrynic acid
- Furosimide

Nonsteroidal anti-inflammatory drugs (NSAIDs)

Quinine derivatives

Causes of Speech Problems

Bilingual caretakers (speech and/or language)

Cerebral palsy

Craniofacial abnormalities

Epileptic aphasia syndrome

Hearing loss
- Pendred syndrome
- Usher syndrome
- Waardenburg syndrome

Juvenile-onset Huntington disease

Maturation delay (developmental language delay)

Mental retardation
- Bardet-Biedl syndrome
- Prader-Willi syndrome
- Williams syndrome

Selective/elective mutism (mixed speech or language delay)

Twin (delay)

Causes of Language Problems

Anemia (severe)

Behavioral problems (may be primary or secondary to speech/language problem)

Cognitive impairment

Deprivation or neglect

Hearing loss

Heavy metals
- Lead
- Mercury

Learning disorders
- Attention deficit disorder/attention deficit hyperactivity disorder (ADD/ADHD)
- Dyslexia

Maturation delay

Mental retardation/developmental delay

Pervasive developmental disorder-autism spectrum

Psychiatric disorders

Specific language impairment

- Expressive language delay
- Mixed
- Receptive language delay

Specific neurodevelopmental syndromes

Key Historical Features

✓ Caregiver, family, or teacher concern about not meeting perceived milestones

✓ Detailed history of developmental milestones at specific ages

✓ Prenatal and birth history
- Maternal health status
- Maternal substance abuse
- Preterm
- Low birth weight
- Infection
- Trauma
- Hypoxia
- Kernicterus

✓ Medical history
- Major illnesses
- Past use of ototoxic medications (aminoglycosides, diuretics, NSAIDs)
- Feeding difficulties
- Recurrent or persistent otitis media
- Seizures
- Severe jaundice
- Trauma
- Endocrine or metabolic disorders

✓ Family history
- Speech or language problems
- Sensorineural hearing loss

✓ Psychosocial history

✓ Number of languages spoken to the child

✓ Aptitude of verbal versus nonverbal communication

✓ Level of intelligence in other areas

✓ Motor development milestones

✓ Language development milestones

✓ Ability of child to communicate with close family members versus strangers or medical team

Key Examination Findings

✓ Plotting of weight, height, and head circumference over time

✓ Vision and hearing evaluations

✓ General evaluation of well-being

✓ Evaluation of appropriate eye contact

✓ Craniofacial examination for anatomic or syndromic abnormalities

✓ Head and neck examination for:

- Cleft lip or palate
- Heterochromia of the irises
- Abnormal anatomy in or around the ears
- Abnormal mobility of the tympanic membrane with pneumatic otoscopy
- Goiter

✓ Thorough neurologic examination

✓ Skin and hair examination for any discoloration

✓ Close observation of parental-child interaction

- Does the child appear anxious away from parents?
- Does the parent answer questions directed toward the child?
- Does the child verbally communicate only with the parent or a close family member?

Suggested Work-Up

Early Language Milestone Scale	Used to assess language development in children younger than 3 years. Focuses on expressive, receptive, and visual language. Relies primarily on the parents' report

Peabody Picture Vocabulary Test Revised	Used for children 2.5 to 18 years of age to screen for word comprehension. If the child is bilingual, performance on the test should be compared with that of other bilingual children of similar cultural and linguistic backgrounds
Denver Developmental Screening Test	Comprehensive developmental assessment to evaluate for a global intellectual impairment, which may manifest initially as a delay in speech development
Audiometry	Indicated for all children with speech delay
Tympanometry	To evaluate eardrum compliance
Complete blood count (CBC) and general chemistry panel	May be considered to screen for anemia or metabolic disorders

Additional Work-Up

Test of intelligence	For children whose results on the Denver Developmental Screening Test indicate an abnormal condition
Auditory brainstem response	Useful in infants and uncooperative children to evaluate for peripheral hearing loss
Karyotype for chromosomal abnormalities and a DNA test	For children who have the phenotypic appearance of fragile X syndrome
Electroencephalogram (EEG)	Should be considered for children with seizures or with significant receptive language disabilities
Thyroid-stimulating hormone (TSH)	If hypothyroidism is suspected
Referral to a pediatric neurologist	If a neurologic disorder is suspected

Referral to a developmental pediatrician	If a developmental delay is suspected or discovered on the Denver Developmental Screening Test

References

1. Coplan J. Quantifying language development from birth to 3 years using the Early Language Milestone Scale. *Pediatrics* 1990;86(6):963–971.

2. Cunningham M, Cox EO. Hearing assessment in infants and children: recommendations beyond neonatal screening. *Pediatrics* 2003;111(2):436–440.

3. Denckla MB. Language disorders. In: Downey JA, Low NL, eds. *The Child with Disabling Illness:Principles of Rehabilitation.* New York: Raven; 1982:175–202.

4. Feldman MH. Evaluation and management of language and speech disorders in preschool children. *Pediatr Rev* 2005;26:131–141.

5. Leung AKC, Kao CP. Evaluation and management of the child with speech delay. *Am Fam Physician* 1999;59:3121–3127.

6. Schum RL. Language screening in the pediatric office setting. *Pediatr Clin North Am* 2007;54(3):425–436.

7. Schwartz ER. Speech and language disorders. In: Schwartz MW, ed. *Pediatric Primary Care: A Problem Oriented Approach.* St. Louis: Mosby; 1990:696–700.

8. Shonkoff JP. Language delay: late talking to communication disorder. In: Rudolph AM, Hoffman JI, Rudolph CD, eds. *Rudolph's Pediatrics.* London: Prentice-Hall; 1996:124–128.

9. U.S. Preventive Services Task Force. Screening for speech and language delay in preschool children: recommendation statement. *Pediatrics* 2006;117:497–501.

10. Yoon G, et al. Speech and language delay are early manifestations of juvenile-onset Huntington disease. *Neurology* 2006;67:1265–1267.

Theodore X. O'Connell

Strabismus refers to ocular misalignment and is one of the most common reasons for referral of pediatric patients to ophthalmologists. Strabismus includes a heterogeneous group of eye movement problems ranging from constant to latent, and from congenital to those acquired late in life. The ocular misalignment present in strabismus interferes with the development and use of normal binocular vision and results in permanent loss of stereopsis (depth perception) if the eyes are not realigned early in development. *Strabismus* may also interfere with the ability to fix visually on objects of regard and to follow moving objects.

Before 6 weeks of age, coordination of eye movements is poor, and the eyes in normal infants may be misaligned. In fact, the eyes of most children are mildly *exotropic* (deviating outward). By the age of 3 months, infants' alignment is stable, and abnormalities of alignment may be diagnosed more accurately. Any strabismus occurring after age 3 months is abnormal.

Infantile strabismus is defined as constant misalignment present before 6 months of age. Infantile strabismus includes *infantile esotropia* (inward deviation) and *exotropia* (ouward deviation).

Infantile esotropia is not always observed at birth but is readily apparent by three months of age. There is frequently a family history of strabismus, and this type of strabismus is not usually associated with any other neurologic or developmental problems. Infants with congenital esotropia must be treated before two years of age for optimal visual outcome. Therefore, early detection and treatment of strabismus are essential to maximize potential visual function. The treatment for infantile esotropia usually consists of surgery to realign the eyes. Early surgical realignment appears to result in better outcomes than does later intervention.

Infantile exotropia is much less common than esotropia and is seen frequently in association with cerebral palsy, prematurity, structural abnormalities in an eye, craniofacial syndromes, and other neurodevelopmental conditions. Any exotropia that occurs after the age of 4 months is abnormal. The treatment of infantile exotropia also consists of surgery to realign the eyes, though the outcomes depend on the associated conditions.

Accommodative esotropia (also known as *acquired esotropia*) occurs after 6 months of life in patients with refractive errors requiring a greater than normal amount of accommodation and in patients with inherently excessive reflexive convergence. This is the most common type of childhood esotropia. Accommodative esotropia appears in children from 6 months to 7 years of age, although it is most common between 2 and 3 years of age. Children with this condition are usually more farsighted than are children without the condition. Treatment consists of glasses to correct refractive error and reduce the need for accommodation. Surgery may be required if other measures do not realign the eyes and also is required for children with esotropia who are not farsighted.

Intermittent exotropia occurs in children after the age of 6 months and occurs when the child looks at distant objects or when the child is fatigued. The eyes may be completely straight when the child looks at near objects. The parents may report observing the child habitually closing the nondominant eye when outdoors. Intermittent exotropia does not routinely require treatment because vision and stereopsis may be normal under usual circumstances. However, patients with more frequent or consistent intermittent exotropia and patients who regress to constant exotropia may require intermittent patching, eyeglasses, vision therapy, or surgery to regain binocular vision.

Pseudoesotropia occurs when the eyes appear crossed as the result of broad epicanthal folds, a wide nasal bridge, or narrow-set eyes. The eyes may appear crossed because of the small amount of sclera that is visible nasally compared with temporally, especially when the child looks to the side. Caution should be exercised in making this diagnosis, however, as true strabismus may coexist with pseudoesotropia.

New-onset strabismus in a school-age child is unusual and warrants neurologic evaluation. Most cases of strabismus in this age group are the result of recurrence of a partially treated strabismus earlier in life.

Causes of Strabismus

Accommodative esotropia

Brown syndrome (congenital or acquired abnormality of the trochlea, resulting in vertical misalignment)

Congenital cranial nerve III palsy

Congenital cranial nerve IV palsy

Congenital cranial nerve VI palsy

Cranial nerve palsies due to other processes

- Arteriovenous malformations
- Diabetes (rare in children)
- Elevated intracranial pressure
- Hypertension (rare in children)
- Infectious, especially viral causes
- Intracranial and orbital masses
- Ischemic
- Trauma

Duane syndrome (congenital aberrant innervation of cranial nerves III and VI)

Infantile esotropia

Infantile exotropia

Intermittent exotropia

Traumatic strabismus associated with orbital fracture

Key Historical Features

✓   Period of onset

✓   Rate of progression, if any

✓   Frequency of strabismus

✓   Amount (amplitude) of deviation

✓   Constancy versus intermittency

✓   Presence or absence of fixation preference (which eye is usually deviated)

✓   Any neurologic symptoms

✓   Past medical history

- Prematurity
- Prenatal drug or alcohol exposure
- Head trauma
- Neurologic disorders
- Cerebral palsy
- Chromosomal or genetic anomalies

✓   Family history of strabismus or amblyopia

Key Physical Findings

✓   Corneal light reflex test. With the infant fixating on the light and the observer directly behind the light, displacement of the light reflex from the center of the pupil demonstrates abnormal alignment of the eyes.

✓   Cover test

✓   Alternate cover test

Suggested Work-Up

Referral to an ophthalmologist is recommended when strabismus is noted in a pediatric patient.

References

1. Donahue SP. Pediatric strabismus. *N Engl J Med* 2007;356:1040–1047.
2. Mills MD. The eye in childhood. *Am Fam Physician* 1999;60:907–918.
3. Ticho BH. Strabismus. *Pediatr Clin North Am* 2003;50:173–188.

Kevin Haggerty

Stridor is defined as turbulent airflow through a narrowed segment of airway or air passages. The word stridor is derived from the Latin "stidere" or "stridulus" signifying to whistle, creak, or make a harsh noise.

Stridor is not a disease; rather, it is a symptom of underlying airway or soft tissue pathology. Although a relatively common finding in pediatric populations, patients presenting with stridor require a prompt and careful evaluation. The patient's age, history, and physical examination findings will provide clues to the underlying cause of stridor.

The most common cause of congenitally acquired stridor is laryngomalacia. Occurring most often in children younger than 2 years of age, laryngomalacia is due to delayed maturation of the structures supporting the airway. The most common cause of acquired stridor is croup, caused by parainfluenza virus. Croup accounts for 80% to 90% of stridor seen in children aged 1 to 4 years. Often croup is accompanied by a characteristic barking or harsh-sounding cough.

Anatomically, stridor is a phenomenon caused by narrowing of the upper airway. The upper airway may be divided into supraglottic, glottic and subglottic, and intrathoracic areas. These anatomic distinctions are essential in targeting the possible causes of stridor (Figure 42-1). The supraglottic area includes the nasopharynx, epiglottis, larynx, aryepiglottic folds, and false vocal cords. The glottic and subglottic area extends from the vocal cords to the extrathoracic portion of the trachea.

Stridor heard on inspiration signals airway obstruction in the supraglottic area. Obstruction in the intrathoracic cavity usually results in stridor that is more pronounced during exhalation. *Biphasic stridor* is the product of obstruction at the glottic or subglottic area, although obstruction in this area may result in inspiratory stridor alone.

Epiglottits, retropharyngeal abcess, and diphtheria infections are among the common causes of inspiratory stridor. Biphasic stidor is most commonly associated with croup, laryngomalacia, or vocal cord paralysis. Stridor that originates from the thorax is most commonly associated with foreign body ingestion.

If a bacterial cause is suspected, rapid and decisive action must be taken.

A patient with an infection of the soft tissue spaces of the neck often will appear toxic and may lie supine with the neck extended in an effort to maintain airway patency. Drooling and the use of the accessory muscles of the neck and abdomen are signs of airway compromise. This patient may require endotracheal intubation or tracheotomy to protect the airway.

Causes of Stridor

Supraglottic Area

- Angioneurotic edema
- Choanal atresia
- Cystic hygroma
- Epiglottitis
- Foreign body
- Gastroesophageal reflux disease
- Hypertrophic tonsils and adenoids
- Intubation (resulting in vocal cord paralysis, laryngotracheal stenosis, subglottic edema, or laryngospasm)
- Laryngeal cyst
- Laryngeal papilloma
- Laryngeal web
- Laryngocele
- Laryngomalacia
- Laryngospasm (hypocalcemic tetany)
- Laryngotracheal stenosis
- Laryngotracheobronchitis (viral croup)
- Lingual thyroid
- Ludwig's angina
- Macroglossia
- Micrognathia
- Peritonsillar abscess
- Psychogenic stridor
- Retropharyngeal abscess
- Subglottic hemangioma
- Thyroglossal cyst
- Vocal cord paralysis

Glottic and Subglottic Area

- Bacterial tracheitis
- External compression of the trachea
  - Anomalous left common carotid artery
  - Lymphadenopathy
  - Lymphoma
  - Mediastinal cyst
  - Right aortic arch with left ligamentum arteriosum

- Gastroesophageal reflux disease (GERD)
- Tracheomalacia
- Vocal cord paralysis

Intrathoracic

- External compression of the trachea
  - o Aberrant subclavian artery
  - o Anomalous innominate artery
  - o Anomalous left pulmonary artery
  - o Double aortic arch
  - o Lymphadenopathy
  - o Lymphoma
  - o Right aortic arch with left ligamentum arteriosum
  - o Teratoma
- Foreign body

Key Historical Features

Age at time of onset (in neonates up to age 6 weeks, congenital abnormalities such as micrognathia, macroglossia, choanal atresia, vocal cord paralysis, laryngeal web, and vascular ring are most likely. Laryngomalacia is the most common cause of chronic stridor in children younger than 2 years. In children aged 1 to 4 years, foreign-body-aspiration and infectious etiologies such as croup and epiglottitis are the most likely causes).

✓ Progression of symptoms

✓ Recent upper respiratory tract infection suggests croup or bacterial tracheitis

✓ Associated symptoms
  - Fever suggests infectious cause
  - Cough suggests croup or tracheal lesion
  - Weak or muffled cry suggests laryngeal anomaly, neuromuscular disorder, or supraglottic lesion
  - Hoarseness suggests vocal cord paralysis or croup
  - Drooling suggests a supraglottic lesion such as abscess, foreign body, or epiglottitis
  - Dysphagia suggests a supraglottic lesion or a foreign body in the trachea
  - Snoring suggests tonsillar or adenoidal hypertrophy

✓ Precipitating factors
  - Worsening at night suggests croup
  - Worsening with feeding suggests tracheoesophageal fistula, tracheomalacia, or a neurologic disorder
  - Worsening with straining or crying suggests laryngomalacia or subglottic hemangioma
  - Worsening in the supine position suggests laryngomalacia, tracheomalacia, or spasmodic cough

✓ Past medical history, especially:
  - Prematurity
  - Complicated delivery
  - Perinatal asphyxia
  - Infection
  - Intubation and mechanical ventilation
  - Cardiac disease
  - Previous admission due to respiratory diseases
  - Atopy

✓ Surgical history, especially:
  - Neck surgery
  - Cardiac surgery
  - Patent ductus arteriosus (PDA) ligation

✓ Family history
  - Down syndrome
  - Hypothyroidism

✓ Social history
  - Exposure to food or environmental allergens
  - Psychosocial stressors

Key Physical Findings

✓ Vital signs, with attention to fever, heart rate, and respiratory rate

✓ Measurement of height and weight

✓ Assessment of potential for impending airway obstruction

✓ General evaluation for evidence of toxicity, cyanosis, respiratory distress, or drooling

✓ Head and neck examination for craniofacial malformation or abnormalities in the size of the tongue or mandible. Examination of the pharynx and soft tissues of the neck for neck edema, lymphadenopathy, or evidence of peritonsillar abscess or pharyngitis. Note any surgical scars on the neck or upper chest.

✓ Observation of the nature and timing of the stridor (inspiratory, expiratory, or biphasic). Note the positioning of the patient and the use of accessory muscles. Note whether the stridor improves when the child is prone.

✓ Auscultation of the mouth and neck to determine the origin of the stridor

✓ Auscultation of the lungs for evidence of abnormal breath sounds

✓ Cardiac examination for murmurs

✓ Extremity examination for clubbing or hemangiomas

✓ Skin examination for café-au-lait spots.

Suggested Work-Up

The most important step in the evaluation of a child with stridor is to determine the degree of airway compromise and the potential for respiratory failure. Prompt airway visualization is essential if epiglottitis or bacterial tracheitis is suspected as the cause of stridor in an acutely ill child. In such cases, airway visualization should be performed by clinicians experienced in managing pediatric airways in a facility equipped with appropriate resuscitation equipment. If the patient does not have a stable airway or needs a thorough evaluation, rigid laryngoscopy, bronchoscopy, or both should be performed in the operating room with anesthesia, sedation, and continuous monitoring.

Complete blood count (CBC)	May be helpful in determining whether an infectious cause is present
Neck radiographs	May reveal changes associated with retropharyngeal abscess (soft tissue air-fluid levels, cervical retroflexion, retropharyngeal space greater than 7 mm anterior to the inferior border of the second cervical vertebral body), croup ("steeple" sign), epiglottitis (thumb sign and a ballooned hypopharyngeal airway), or foreign body (if radio-opaque)

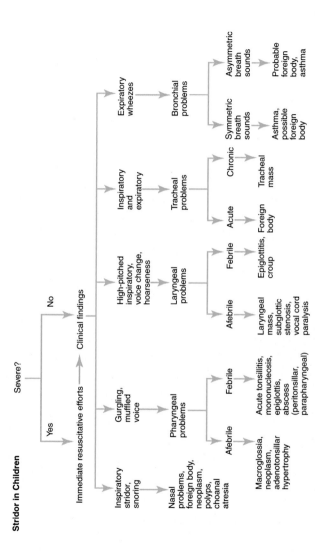

Figure 42-1. Algorithm, based on clinical findings, for evaluating stridor in children. (Adapted with permission from Handler SD. Stridor. In: Fleisher GR, Ludwig S, eds. *Textbook of Pediatric Emergency Medicine.* Baltimore: Williams & Wilkins; 1993:474–478.)

Additional Work-Up

Chest radiographs	If an intrathoracic etiology is suspected
Viral serologies	May be used for confirmatory testing for suspected parainfluenza, influenza A and B, and respiratory syncitial virus infections
Blood cultures	Should be considered in cases of peritonsillar or retropharyngeal abscess
Computed tomography (CT) scan of the neck and chest	May be helpful in diagnosing retropharyngeal abscess and for looking for enlarged lymph nodes, tumor, aberrant arteries, and vascular rings
Magnetic resonance imaging (MRI)	Can be useful in evaluating the trachea and the mediastinum
Airway fluoroscopy	If tracheomalacia is suspected
Barium swallow	May help to identify esophageal abnormalities, GERD, swallowing dysfunction, mediastinal masses, and vascular rings
Gastrograffin swallow	Used instead of barium swallow if tracheoesophageal fistula is suspected
Spirometry	In children older than 6 years, spirometry may be used to help distinguish the site of the obstruction and its response to bronchodilators

References

1. Clark J. The wheezing child. *Clin Pediatr* 2008;47(2):191–198.
2. Friedberg J. An approach to stridor in infants and children. *J Otolaryngol* 1987;16:203–206.
3. Handler SD. Stridor. In: Fleisher GR, Ludwig S, eds. *Textbook of Pediatric Emergency Medicine*. Baltimore: Williams & Wilkins; 1993:474–478.
4. Leung AKC, Cho H. Diagnosis of stridor in children. *Am Fam Physician* 1999;60:2289.
5. Mancuso RF. Stridor in neonates. *Pediatr Clin North Am* 1996;43:1339–1356.
6. Nicklaus PJ, Kelley PE. Management of deep neck infection. *Pediatr Clin North Am* 1996;43(6):1277–1296.
7. Simon NP. Evaluation and management of stridor in the newborn. *Clin Pediatr* 1991;30:211–216.

43 SYNCOPE

Theodore X. O'Connell

Syncope is a sudden, unexpected loss of consciousness associated with a loss of postural tone with spontaneous recovery. A *syncopal event* is one of the more dramatic and anxiety-provoking symptoms encountered by patients, and it often produces a diagnostic dilemma for the clinician. Syncope is a common manifestation of numerous disorders with a final common pathway of insufficient cerebral blood flow to maintain consciousness. Syncope must be differentiated from other disorders of altered consciousness, including seizures, sleep disorders, metabolic disorders, vertigo, presyncope, and psychiatric disorders.

In the evaluation of syncope, proving a specific diagnosis is often difficult because of a lack of residual abnormalities on examination or on initial diagnostic studies. The clinician must remember that syncope is a symptom, not a disease. By possessing an understanding of the common causes of syncope, the clinician can focus the history, physical examination, and diagnostic evaluation in each case. An understanding of the available diagnostic tests and their indications is imperative.

As many as 15% of children and adolescents will have a syncopal event between the ages of 8 and 18 years. Before age 6 years, syncope is unusual except in the setting of seizure disorders, breath-holding, and primary cardiac dysrhythmias. The cause of most cases of syncope can be placed into one of five categories: (1) autonomic, (2) cardiac, (3) psychiatric, (4) neurologic/cerebrovascular, and (5) metabolic/endocrine. Pediatric and young patients are most likely to have *neurocardiogenic syncope* (vasovagal syncope), psychiatric causes, and primary arrhythmic causes such as long QT syndrome and Wolff-Parkinson-White syndrome. The most common type of syncope in otherwise healthy children is *vasovagal syncope*. In infants who have recurrent and severe episodes of syncope that only have their onset in the presence of a particular parent or guardian, factitious or induced illness should be considered.

According to the American Heart Association, the differential diagnosis and evaluation of syncope in pediatric patients are similar to those in adults. The goal of the evaluation is to identify high-risk patients with underlying heart disease, which may include identifiable genetic abnormalities such as the long QT syndrome, Brugada syndrome, or hypertrophic cardiomyopathy.

Syncope associated with high-intensity physical activity is a typical presentation of hypertrophic cardiomyopathy or catecholaminergic polymorphic ventricular tachycardia and generally is evaluated with an electrocardiogram (ECG), echocardiogram, and an exercise stress test. Neurocardiogenic syncope is a common disturbance in the healthy child or adolescent. Breath-holding spells resulting from emotional upset have been reported in 2% to 5% of well patients.

Many algorithms exist for the evaluation of syncope, and most emphasize the importance of the history and physical examination in making an accurate diagnosis. Although algorithms may provide a guide for the evaluation of syncope, the various available algorithms each contain controversial elements. In addition, algorithms do not consider every clinical situation and are not designed to replace individual clinician judgment. The physician should understand the approach to the patient with syncope first and then consult algorithms to focus the diagnostic evaluation.

Medications Associated with Syncope

- α-agonists
- Anticholinergic agents
- Antiparkinsonian agents
- Antipsychotics
- β-adrenergic blockers
- Narcotics
- Vasodilators

Causes of Syncope

Reflex Mediated

- Vasovagal
- Situational (cough, defecation, micturition, swallow)
- Carotid sinus hypersensitivity

Cardiac

- Arrhythmia
- Hypertrophic cardiomyopathy
- Left ventricular outflow tract obstruction
- Myocarditis
- Pulmonary hypertension
- Tamponade
- Tumor or mass
- Valvular disease

Medication Effects

Metabolic Disorders

- Adrenal failure

Hypoglycemia

Neurologic Causes

- Migraine headache (syncopal migraine)
- Transient ischemic attack

Orthostatic Hypotension (Autonomic Dysfunction)

- Amyloidosis
- Diabetes
- Guillain-Barré syndrome
- Human immunodeficiency virus (HIV) infection
- Paraneoplastic neuropathies
- Parkinson's disease
- Shy-Drager syndrome

Psychiatric Causes

- Hyperventilation
- Major depression
- Panic disorder
- Pseudoseizures

Other Causes

- Breath-holding
- Hyperventilation
- Hypovolemia
- Seizure (not a true case of syncope)
- Subclavian steal syndrome

Unknown

Key Historical Features

✓ Situation in which syncope occurred (on standing, in a fearful situation, during micturition, with coughing, with exertion)

✓ Activities leading up to the event

✓ Prodromal symptoms (lightheadedness, warmth, nausea, sweating)

✓ Associated cardiac symptoms (chest pain, palpitations, shortness of breath)

✓ Associated neurologic symptoms (focal neurologic symptoms, headache, diplopia)

✓ Witnessed events (tonic/clonic movements, tongue biting, urinary incontinence)

✓ If witnessed, characterization of the patient's appearance during and immediately following the episode

✓ Duration of the episode

✓ Time of day

✓ Time of last meal

✓ Previous history of syncope

✓ Recent dehydration

✓ Post-event symptoms
  • Confusion may indicate seizure activity
  • Injuries related to a fall
  • Duration of recovery

✓ Medical history, particularly:
  • History of cardiac disease, including coronary artery disease, arrhythmias, or cardiomyopathy
  • History of cerebrovascular ischemia
  • History of pulmonary embolism or pulmonary hypertension
  • History of gastrointestinal (GI) bleeding

✓ Family history of syncope or sudden death

✓ Medications
  • Especially antihypertensive agents, antidepressants, vasodilators, narcotic analgesics, Q-T prolonging agents (tricyclic antidepressants), and hypoglycemic agents

✓ Social history
  • Alcohol or marijuana use
  • Smoking history, which places the patient at risk for cardiopulmonary disease

Key Physical Findings

✓ Vitals signs

✓ Evaluation for orthostatic hypotension (defined as a decrease of at least 20 mm Hg systolic or 10 mm Hg diastolic blood pressure within 3 minutes of standing)

✓ Funduscopic examination

✓   Cardiovascular examination

- Carotid bruits
- Murmurs
- Jugular venous distention
- Loud S2
- Presence of an S3
- Pericardial friction rubs
- Blood pressures in both arms

✓   Neurologic evaluation

- Mental status
- Pupil symmetry
- Evaluation for nystagmus
- Gait evaluation
- Balance and cerebellar function
- Romberg's sign
- Deep tendon reflexes
- Proprioception

Suggested Work-Up

ECG	To identify abnormalities that may suggest an underlying cardiac cause for the syncope. Important findings include a long QT interval, pre-excitation, evidence of conduction disorders, signs of coronary artery disease, or left ventricular hypertrophy that may be associated with ventricular tachycardia
Complete blood count (CBC), electrolytes, blood urea nitrogen (BUN), creatinine, and glucose	Indicated when an underlying disorder is suspected as a potential cause of syncope
Pregnancy test	Should be considered in adolescent females

Additional Work-Up

Cardiology consultation and echocardiogram	Should be obtained if a heart murmur is appreciated, a family history of sudden death or cardiomyopathy exists, or the ECG is at all suspicious

Holter monitoring or telemetry monitoring	Should be considered in patients with a history of palpitations associated with syncope. Also recommended for patients with known or suspected cardiac disease or a suspected arrhythmic cause of syncope
Treadmill exercise stress test	Should be considered if the syncopal event is associated with exercise
Tilt-table testing	May be useful in patients with recurrent unexplained syncope with a suspected neurocardiogenic cause. May also be useful in patients without cardiac disease or in whom cardiac testing has been negative
Cardiac catheterization and electrophysiologic testing	May be indicated for patients with primary dysrhythmias and patients with pre-excitation syndromes such as Wolff-Parkinson-White syndrome and in patients with a suspected bradyarrhythmic cause for syncope
Electroencephalogram (EEG) and neurologic consultation	Indicated in patients exhibiting prolonged loss of consciousness, seizure activity, and a postictal phase of lethargy or confusion. EEG is indicated only when seizure is suspected because the positive yield of EEG is otherwise very low.
24-hour Holter monitor or a loop-recording event monitor	May be useful in patients with a history of palpitations associated with syncope to help capture the cardiac rhythm
Computed tomography (CT)	CT scanning of the head has a relatively low yield in patients with syncope and is not routinely indicated. It is recommended in patients with focal neurologic symptoms and signs. It may be performed in patients with seizure activity and head trauma to rule out intracranial hemorrhage

Psychiatric evaluation	Recommended for patients with recurrent unexplained syncope if there is no cardiac disease or if the cardiac evaluation is negative. Young patients and patients with many prodromal symptoms are at higher risk of having an underlying psychiatric disease associated with their episodes of syncope
Admission to the hospital for observation with continuous ambulatory ECG and EEG monitoring	May be indicated if syncope is reported to be occurring several times a day every day. Video surveillance may be included if factitious or induced illness is suspected

References

1. Abboud FM. Neurocardiogenic syncope. *N Engl J Med* 1993;328:1117–1120.
2. Atkins D, et al. Syncope and orthostatic hypotension. *Am J Med* 1991;91:179–185.
3. Calkins H. Pharmacologic approaches to therapy for vasovagal syncope. *Am J Cardiol* 1999;84:20Q–25Q.
4. Cunningham R, Mikhail MG. Management of patients with syncope and cardiac arrhythmias in an emergency department observation unit. *Emerg Med Clin North Am* 2001;19:105–121.
5. Davis TL, Freemon FR. Electroencephalography should not be routine in the evaluation of syncope in adults. *Arch Inter Med* 1990;150:2027–2029.
6. Di Girolamo E, et al. Effects of paroxetine hydrochloride, a selective serotonin reuptake inhibitor, on refractory vasovagal syncope: a randomized, double-blind, placebo-controlled study. *J Am Coll Cardiol* 1999;33:1227–1230.
7. Kaufmann H. Neurally mediated syncope: pathogenesis, diagnosis, and treatment. *Neurology* 1995;45(suppl 5):S12–S18.
8. Kapoor WN. Syncope. *N Engl J Med* 2000;343:1856–1862.
9. Kelly AM, et al. Breath-holding spells associated with significant bradycardia; successful treatment with permanent pacemaker implantation. *Pediatrics* 2001;108:698–702.
10. Lewis DA, Dhala A. Syncope in the pediatric patient: the cardiologist's perspective. *Pediatr Clin North Am* 1999;46:205–219.
11. Linzer M, et al. Diagnosing syncope, Part 1: value of history, physical examination and electrocardiography. Clinical efficacy assessment project of the American College of Physicians. *Ann Intern Med* 1997;126:989–996.
12. Linzer M, et al. Diagnosing syncope, Part 2: unexplained syncope. Clinical efficacy project of the American College of Physicians. *Ann Intern Med* 1997;127:76–86.
13. Mahananda N, et al. Randomized double-blind, placebo-controlled trial of oral atenolol in patients with unexplained syncope and positive upright tilt table test results. *Am Heart J* 1995;130:1250–1253.
14. McLeod KA. Syncope in childhood. *Arch Dis Child* 2003;88:350–353.
15. Munro NC, et al. Incidence of complications after carotid sinus massage in older patients with syncope. *J Am Geriatr Soc* 1994;42:1248–1251.
16. Rodriguez-Nunez A, et al. Cerebral syncope in children. *J Pediatr* 2000;136:542–544.

17. Sapin SO. Autonomic syncope in pediatrics: a practice-oriented approach to classification, pathophysiology, diagnosis, and management. *Clin Pediatr* 2004;43:17–23.

18. Schnipper JL, Kapoor WN. Diagnostic evaluation and management of patients with syncope. *Med Clin North Am* 2001;85:423–456.

19. Strckberger SA, et al. AHA/ACCF scientific statement on the evaluation of syncope: from the American Heart Association Councils on Clinical Cardiology, Cardiovascular Nursing, Cardiovascular Disease in the Young, and Stroke, and the Quality Care and Outcomes Research Interdisciplinary Working Group; and the American College of Cardiology Foundation: in collaboration with the Heart Rhythm Society: endorsed by the American Autonomic Society. *Circulation* 2006;113:316–327.

20. Sutton R, et al. Dual chamber pacing in the treatment of neurally mediated positive cardioinhibitory syncope: pacemaker versus no therapy—a multicenter randomized study. The Vasovagal Syncope International Study (VASIS) Investigators. *Circulation* 2000;102:294–299.

21. Sutton R, et al. Proposed classification for tilt induced vasovagal syncope. *Eur J Pacing Electrophysiol* 1992;3:180–183.

22. Ward CR, et al. Midodrine: a role in the management of neurocardiogenic syncope. *Heart* 1998;79:45–49.

23. Weimer LH. Syncope and orthostatic intolerance for the primary care physician. *Primary Care Clin Office Pract* 2004;31:175–199.

24. Zeng C, et al. Randomized, double-blind, placebo-controlled trial of oral enalapril in patients with neurally mediated syncope. *Am Heart J* 1998;136:852–858.

25. Zimetbaum P, et al. Utility of patient-activated cardiac event recorders in general clinical practice. *Am J Cardiol* 1997;79:371–372.

Theodore X. O'Connell

Normal platelet counts in children and term infants are 150,000 to 450,000/μL of blood. Normal platelet counts in preterm infants are in this same range but tend to average on the lower end of normal. *Thrombocytopenia* is defined as a platelet count of less than 150,000/μL of blood.

Idiopathic (immune) thrombocytopenic purpura (ITP) is the most common cause of thrombocytopenia in childhood and usually occurs in children between the ages of 2 and 4 years. In about 90% of children with ITP, the disease is an acute, self-limited process that usually resolves within 6 months. Chronic ITP is more common in children older than 10 years and in those younger than 1 year of age. In ITP, the complete blood count (CBC) will show an isolated thrombocytopenia with normal white (WBC) and red blood cell (RBC) counts. Examination of the peripheral smear is important to evaluate platelet size, WBC differential and morphology, RBC morphology, and to rule out the presence of microangiopathic changes such as schistocytes, which might suggest another diagnosis. If the history, physical examination, CBC, and peripheral smear are normal except for thrombocytopenia, a bone marrow biopsy may be deferred.

Neonatal thrombocytopenia is relatively common, occurring in 2% to 3% of healthy term infants and 20% to 30% of all sick neonates. In general, the thrombocytopenia seen in a sick infant is likely related to the primary disease process and resolves as the primary process improves.

Neonatal alloimmune thrombocytopenia occurs in 1 in 1000 births. The typical presentation is that of a full-term infant who is otherwise healthy, born after an uncomplicated pregnancy and delivery, and found to have petechiae or bruising on examination and confirmed to have a significant degree of thrombocytopenia. The thrombocytopenia is caused by transplacental passage of maternal alloantibodies directed against fetal platelet antigens inherited from the father but absent on maternal platelets. This process is the platelet equivalent of Rh-hemolytic disease of the newborn. In contrast to Rh-hemolytic disease of the newborn, neonatal alloimmune thrombocytopenia often develops in the first pregnancy of an at-risk couple.

The thrombocytopenia seen in autoimmune thrombocytopenia is less severe than in alloimmune thrombocytopenia, with only 10% to 15% of patients having a neonatal platelet count less than 50,000/μL. As such, autoimmune thrombocytopenia is associated with a lower bleeding rate. The history will reveal a low maternal platelet count, maternal ITP, or possibly maternal systemic lupus erythematosus (SLE) or hypothyroidism. All neonates of mothers with autoimmune disease should be considered for cord blood platelet count at birth and again at 24 hours to evaluate for thrombocytopenia. In affected children, spontaneous recovery of the platelet count usually occurs within 3 weeks after birth.

If the history and physical examination are not suggestive of thrombocytopenia, pseudothrombocytopenia or "artifactual" thrombocytopenia should be considered. The platelet count can be repeated using a citrated tube to assess the count in the absence of platelet clumping.

Medications Associated with Thrombocytopenia

- Alkylating agents
- Anti-arrhythmic drugs
- Anticonvulsants
- Antimetabolites
- Chlorothiazide diuretics
- Cimetidine
- Estrogens
- H_2 antagonists
- Heparin
- Nitrofurantoin
- Nonsteroidal anti-inflammatory drugs (NSAIDs)
- Penicillin
- Quinidine
- Sulfonamides
- Ticlopidine
- Valproic acid

Causes of Thrombocytopenia

Neonatal

Alloimmune thrombocytopenia

Asphyxia

Congenital and inherited causes

- Amegakarocytic thrombocytopenia
- Autosomal dominant thrombocytopenia
- Bernard-Soulier syndrome
- Chediak-Higashi syndrome
- Congenital leukemia
- Fanconi's anemia
- Fechtner syndrome
- Kasabach-Merritt syndrome
- May-Hegglin anomaly

- Montreal syndrome
- Quebec platelet disorder
- Sebastian syndrome
- Thrombocytopenia absent radius (TAR) syndrome
- Triploidy
- Trisomy 13
- Trisomy 18
- Trisomy 21
- Wiskott-Aldrich syndrome
- X-linked thrombocytopenia

Congenital infection

- Cytomegalovirus (CMV)
- Human immunodeficiency virus (HIV)
- Rubella
- *Toxoplasma* spp.

Disseminated intravascular coagulation (DIC)

Maternal idiopathic (immune) thrombocytopenia purpura

Metabolic disease

- Methylmalonic acidemia
- Proprionic acidemia

Necrotizing enterocolitis

Neonatal cold injury

Perinatal infection

- *Escherichia coli*
- Guillain-Barré syndrome
- *Haemophilus influenzae*

Placental insufficiency

Pregnancy-induced hypertension

Respiratory distress syndrome (RDS)

Rh hemolytic disease (severe)

Sepsis

Thrombosis of aortic or renal vein

Childhood

Aplastic anemia

Autoimmune disease

- Juvenile rheumatoid arthritis (RA)
- SLE

Bone marrow infiltration

- Granulomatous diseases
- Histiocytosis
- Leukemia
- Myelofibrosis
- Storage disorders

Disseminated intravascular coagulation

Drug induced thrombocytopenia

Fanconi anemia

Hemangioma

Hemolytic uremic syndrome

ITP

Immunodeficiencies

May-Hegglin anomaly

Thrombotic thrombocytopenia purpura

Type 2 von Willebrand disease

Key Historical Features

✓ Onset and duration of bruising or bleeding

✓ Location of bleeding

✓ Antecedent viral infection

✓ Fever

✓ Weight loss

✓ Bone pain

✓ Joint pain

✓ Abdominal pain

✓ Blood in stools

✓ Hematuria

✓ Menometrorrhagia

✓ Epistaxis

✓ Medical history

✓ Birth history

✓ Maternal history if thrombocytopenia has neonatal onset

✓ Past surgical history

✓ Medications

✓ Family history of bleeding disorder

Key Physical Findings

✓ Vital signs, noting fever or hypertension

✓ Growth parameters and comparison with previous measurements

✓ General evaluation of well-being

✓ Complete skin examination for purpura, pallor, rash, jaundice, café-au-lait spots, or telangiectasias

✓ Evaluation for lymphadenopathy

✓ Abdominal examination for tenderness or hepatosplenomegaly

✓ Genitourinary examination for scrotal edema

✓ Extremity examination for edema, palmar erythema, or evidence of hemarthrosis

Suggested Work-Up

CBC with differential	To measure the platelet count and evaluate the other blood cell lines
Peripheral smear	To evaluate platelet size, WBC differential and morphology, RBC morphology, and to rule out the presence of microangiopathic changes such as schistocytes, which might suggest another diagnosis
Coombs' test	If an autoimmune-mediated thrombocytopenia is suspected
Antigen testing of mother's and father's platelets with testing of mother's serum for antiplatelet alloantibody	If neonatal alloimmune thrombocytopenia is suspected
Transcranial ultrasound	Indicated in all severely thrombocytopenic (<30,000/μL) neonates to evaluate for intracranial hemorrhage

Prothrombin time, activated partial thromboplastin time, plasma fibrinogen concentration, fibrin degradation product, D-dimer	If disseminated intravascular coagulation (DIC) is suspected. In DIC, prothrombin time is prolonged, activated partial thromboplastin time is prolonged, plasma fibrinogen concentration is decreased, fibrin degradation product is increased, and D-dimer is elevated

Additional Work-Up

Identification and treatment of the underlying cause is indicated if a primary disease process is suspected in cases of neonatal thrombocytopenia. Infants who appear ill should be evaluated for sepsis. Evaluation for congenital infection or genetic testing may be indicated.

Bone marrow examination	Indicated for any child with thrombocytopenia with an atypical presentation or with thrombocytopenia lasting for longer than 6 months to evaluate for other conditions that could result in thrombocytopenia
Maternal platelet count	To distinguish alloimmune thrombocytopenia from autoimmune thrombocytopenia

References

1. Bolton-Maggs HB. Idiopathic thrombocytopenic purpura. *Arch Dis Child* 2000;83:220–222.
2. Cines DB, Blanchette VS. Immune thrombocytopenic purpura. *N Engl J Med* 2002;346: 995–1008.
3. Kaplan RN, Bussel JB. Differential diagnosis and management of thrombocytopenia in childhood. *Pediatr Clin North Am* 2004;51:1109–1140.
4. Roberts I, Murray NA. Neonatal thrombocytopenia: causes and management. *Arch Dis Child Fetal Neonatal Educ* 2003;88:359–364.

Theodore X. O'Connell

The first step in the evaluation of transaminase elevation is to repeat the test to confirm the result. Both alanine aminotransferase (ALT) and aspartate aminotransferase (AST) are released into the blood in increasing amounts when the liver cell membrane is damaged. However, necrosis of liver cells is not required for the release of the aminotransferases, and correlation between the level of the aminotransferases and the degree of liver cell damage is poor.

The initial evaluation includes a detailed history, review of medications, and a physical examination. The history should include an assessment of the patient's risk factors for liver disease with attention directed toward family history, medications, vitamins, herbal supplements, alcohol consumption, drug use, history of blood-product transfusions, and symptoms of liver disease. Signs of liver disease are outlined below.

Common causes of elevated aminotransferase levels are alcohol-related liver injury, hepatitis B and C, autoimmune hepatitis, fatty infiltration of the liver, nonalcoholic steatohepatitis (NASH), hemochromatosis, Wilson's disease, alpha$_1$-antitrypsin deficiency, and celiac disease. Alcohol-related liver injury is a common cause of elevated aminotransferase levels and must be considered in any child or adolescent who may be drinking.

The term NASH was first used in 1980 in describing 20 nonalcoholic patients with liver biopsy changes compatible with alcoholic hepatitis. NASH may be considered part of a larger spectrum of nonalcoholic fatty liver disorders (NAFLD) that extends from simple steatosis through NASH. Liver biopsy is necessary for definitive diagnosis of NASH, which is characterized by fatty change with lobular inflammation, hepatocellular injury, and Mallory hyaline, with or without fibrosis, in the absence of excessive alcohol consumption. In contrast, simple fatty liver is characterized histologically by hepatic steatosis without inflammation, ballooning degeneration, necrosis, fibrosis, or cirrhosis.

Recent studies suggest that NASH may not be rare in children, especially in obese children, and severe fibrosis may be found at an early age. Therefore, NASH should be considered in obese children with elevated aminotransferase levels. Liver biopsy is the gold standard for the diagnosis of NAFLD/NASH to confirm the diagnosis and establish severity of fibrosis and the presence of cirrhosis. Liver biopsy also excludes other coexisting conditions that can result in hepatic steatosis.

Medications That May Cause Transaminase Elevation

- Acetaminophen
- Amiodarone

- Amoxicillin-clavulanic acid
- Aspirin
- Azathioprine/6-MP
- Carbamazepine
- Ciprofloxacin
- Cyclosporine
- Erythromycin
- Estrogens
- Fluconazole
- Glipizide
- Glucocorticoids
- Glyburide
- Halothane
- Heparin
- Isoniazid
- Ketoconazole
- L-asparaginase
- Labetalol
- Methotrexate
- Minocycline
- Nitrofurantoin
- Nonsteroidal anti-inflammatory drugs (NSAIDs)
- Pemoline
- Phenobarbital
- Phenytoin
- Propylthiouracil
- Protease inhibitors
- Statin medications
- Sulfonamides
- Synthetic penicillins
- Trazodone
- Valproic acid

Causes of Transaminitis

Acquired muscle diseases
Acute viral hepatitis
Alcohol

Alpha$_1$-antitrypsin deficiency

Autoimmune hepatitis

Celiac disease

Chronic hepatitis B

Chronic hepatitis C

Cirrhosis

Cystic fibrosis

Diabetes, especially type 1

Hemochromatosis

Hemolysis

Hyperthyroidism

Inborn errors of metabolism

- Abetalipoproteinemia
- Carnitine deficiency
- Fatty acid oxidation
- Glycogen storage
- Organic acidemia
- Urea cycle

Inherited disorders of muscle metabolism

Jejuno-ileal bypass

Medications

NASH

Nonprescription medications

- Alchemilla
- Anabolic steroids
- Chaparral leaf
- Cocaine
- Ephedra (mahuang)
- Gentian
- Germander
- Glues containing toluene
- Jin bu huan
- Kava
- MDMA ("ecstasy")
- Phencyclidine
- Scutellaria (skullcap)
- Senna
- Shark cartilage

- Trichloroethylene
- Vitamin A

Nutritional deficiency (starvation, rapid weight loss, kwashiorkor)

Steatosis

Strenuous exercise

Syndromes associated with insulin resistance

- Bardet-Biedl syndrome
- Lipodystrophy syndromes
- Prader-Willi syndrome

Wilson's disease (in patients younger than 40 years old)

Key Historical Features

✓ Abdominal pain

✓ Anorexia

✓ Malaise

✓ Nausea and vomiting

✓ Systemic features of drug hypersensitivity
  - Fever
  - Rash

✓ Use of parenteral nutrition

✓ Rapid weight loss

✓ Past medical history

✓ Past surgical history, especially intestinal or biliary surgery

✓ Medications

✓ Vitamins

✓ Herbal supplements

✓ Family medical history

✓ Social history
  - Alcohol use
  - Drug use

Key Physical Findings

✓ Acanthosis nigricans

✓ Ascites

✓ Bleeding problems

✓ Caput medusae

✓ Features suggesting confounding syndromes

- Deafness
- Dysmorphic facies
- Hypotonia
- Neurodevelopmental delay
- Retinal dystrophy
- Short stature

✓ Gynecomastia

✓ Hemorrhoids

✓ Impotence

✓ Jaundice

✓ Liver size

✓ Mental status changes

✓ Palmar erythema

✓ Spider angiomata

✓ Splenomegaly

✓ Testicular atrophy

Suggested Work-Up

ALT, AST	AST:ALT ratio >2 suggests alcohol abuse AST:ALT ratio <1 suggests NASH
Total and direct bilirubin, alkaline phosphatase, gamma-glutamyl transpeptidase (GGT)	To evaluate biliary excretion
Prothrombin time	To assess hepatic synthetic function
Albumin	To assess hepatic synthetic function
Complete blood count (CBC)	To evaluate for infection, neutropenia, thrombocytopenia
Fasting serum glucose and insulin level	To evaluate for insulin resistance
Fasting lipid panel	To evaluate for hyperlipidemia

Hepatitis C antibody	To evaluate for hepatitis C infection
Hepatitis B surface antigen, surface antibody, and core antibody	To evaluate for hepatitis B infection
Serum iron, ferritin, and total iron-binding capacity	Iron overload suggests hemochromatosis
Serum ceruloplasmin	Decreased level suggests Wilson disease
α_1-antitrypsin phenotyping	To evaluate for α_1-antitrypsin deficiency
Gliadin and endomesial antibodies	Immunoglobulin A (IgA) antibodies to both gliadin and endomysium are 95% sensitive and specific for the diagnosis of celiac disease
Urine organic acids and serum amino acids	To evaluate for inborn errors of metabolism (particularly important in children who are not obese and are presenting at a younger age)

Additional Work-Up (May Be Indicated If Above Tests Are Normal)

Chloride sweat test	If cystic fibrosis is suspected
Hepatitis A immunoglobulins	If hepatitis A infection is suspected on the basis of history and physical examination
Cytomegalovirus (CMV) immunoglobulins	If CMV infection is suspected
Epstein-Barr virus immunoglobulins	If Epstein-Barr virus is suspected
Acetaminophen and aspirin levels	If toxicity or overdose is suspected
Quantitative hepatitis C virus ribonucleic acid (RNA)	If hepatitis C antibody is positive
Liver ultrasonography	To evaluate for hepatic steatosis, cholelithiasis, cholecystitis evidence of cirrhosis, or a liver mass

Liver biopsy	May be indicated to exclude other diseases and to help make a specific diagnosis

References

1. American Gastroenterological Association. Medical position statement: evaluation of liver chemistry tests. *Gastroenterology* 2002;123:1364–1366.
2. Davison S. Celiac disease and liver dysfunction. *Arch Dis Child* 2002;87:293–296.
3. Giboney PT. Mildly elevated liver transaminase levels in the asymptomatic patient. *Am Fam Physician* 2005;71:1105–10.
4. Green RM, Flamm S. AGA technical review on the evaluation of liver chemistry tests. *Gastroenterology* 2002;123:1367–1384.
5. Kumar KS, Malet PF. Nonalcoholic steatohepatitis. *Mayo Clin Proc* 2000;75:733–739.
6. Lavine JE, Schwimmer JB. Nonalcoholic fatty liver disease in the pediatric population. *Clin Liver Dis* 2004;8:549–558.
7. Ludwig J, Viggiano TR, McGill DB, Ott BJ. Nonalcoholic steatohepatitis: Mayo Clinic experiences with a hitherto unnamed disease. *Mayo Clin Proc* 1980;55:434–438.
8. Marion AW, Baker AJ, Dhawan A. Fatty liver disease in children. *Arch Dis Child* 2004;89:648–652.
9. Pineiro-Carrero VM, Pineiro EO. Liver. *Pediatrics* 2004;113:1097–1106.
10. Pratt DS, Kaplan MM. Evaluation of abnormal liver enzyme results in asymptomatic patients. *N Engl J Med* 2000;342:1266–1271.
11. Swartz MH. *Textbook of Physical Diagnosis*, 2nd ed. Philadelphia: WB Saunders; 1994: 302–336.

Theodore X. O'Connell

Urinary tract infection (UTI) in the pediatric population is well recognized as a cause of acute morbidity. Children with vesicoureteral reflux (VUR) are believed to be at risk for ongoing renal damage with subsequent infections, resulting in hypertension and renal insufficiency in adulthood. Infants and young children are at higher risk than are older children for incurring acute renal injury with UTI. The incidence of VUR is higher in this age group than in older children, and the severity of VUR is greater. The risk of renal damage increases as the number of recurrences increases.

The American Academy of Pediatrics 1999 Practice Parameter focuses on the diagnosis, treatment, and evaluation of febrile infants and young children 2 months to 2 years of age. Children older than 2 years were excluded because they are more likely than younger children to have symptoms referable to the urinary tract, are less likely to have factors predisposing them to renal damage, and are at lower risk of developing renal damage.

During the first year of life, boys have a higher incidence of UTI; in all other age groups, girls are more prone to developing UTI. Up to 7% of girls and 2% of boys will have a symptomatic, culture-confirmed UTI by 6 years of age. Most UTIs in children result from ascending infections, although hematogenous spread may be more common in the first 12 weeks of life. *Escherichia coli* (*E. coli*) is the most frequent documented uropathogen. Among neonates, UTI attributable to group B streptococcus is more common than in older populations.

Children who have UTI often do not show the characteristic signs and symptoms seen in the adult population. Older children with UTI may have dysuria, urgency, frequency, or lower abdominal pain. Infants with UTI more commonly present with nonspecific symptoms such as fever, irritability, vomiting, failure to thrive (FTT), or jaundice. The presence of UTI should be considered in infants and young children 2 months to 2 years of age with unexplained fever. The prevalence of UTI in children of this age who have no fever source evident from the history or physical examination is about 5%.

Diagnosis of UTI requires a culture of the urine, which must be properly collected. Urinalysis can only suggest the diagnosis. In infants and young children 2 months to 2 years of age, the urine specimen should be obtained by suprapubic aspiration or transurethral bladder catheterization. The diagnosis of UTI cannot be established by a culture of urine collected in a bag. Older children can provide a clean-catch midstream urine specimen.

Imaging of the urinary tract is recommended in every febrile infant or young child with a first UTI to identify those with abnormalities that predispose to renal damage. Imaging consists of urinary tract ultrasonography to identify hydronephrosis, dilatation of the distal ureters, hypertrophy of the bladder wall, and the presence of ureteroceles. In addition, either voiding cystourethrography (VCUG) or radionuclide cystography (RNC) is recommended for detecting reflux.

Initial antimicrobial therapy should be administered parenterally, and hospitalization should be considered for the infant or child with suspected UTI who is assessed as toxic, dehydrated, or unable to retain oral intake. For the infant or child who does not appear ill but who has a culture confirming the presence of UTI, antimicrobial therapy should be initiated either parenterally or orally. Seven to 14 days of oral antimicrobial therapy should be completed. Children 2 months to 2 years of age with UTI should receive antimicrobials in therapeutic or prophylactic dosages until the imaging studies are completed to prevent recurrent infection.

If a child does not have the expected clinical response within 2 days of antimicrobial therapy, the child should be reevaluated and another urine specimen should be cultured. Children who do not respond clinically should undergo ultrasonography promptly. In addition, either VCUG or RNC should be performed at the earliest convenient time.

Risk Factors for Pediatric Urinary Tract Infections

Anatomic Abnormalities

- Posterior urethral valves
- Vesicoureteral reflux

Fecal and Perineal Colonization

Functional Abnormalities

- Neurogenic bladder

Gender

Immunocompromised States

Neonates and Infants

Sexual Activity

Uncircumcised Status (During the First Year of Life)

Key Historical Features

✓ Onset of symptoms

✓ Fever

✓ Crying on urination

✓ Altered voiding pattern

✓ Dysuria

✓   Urgency

✓   Urinary frequency

✓   Hesitancy

✓   Oliguria

✓   Vomiting

✓   Anorexia

✓   Irritability

✓   Lethargy

✓   Malodorous urine

✓   Jaundice

✓   FTT

✓   Birth history

✓   Past medical history

✓   Past surgical history

Key Physical Findings

✓   Vital signs

✓   General assessment of well-being

✓   Back examination for costovertebral angle tenderness

✓   Abdominal examination for suprapubic tenderness

✓   Sacral examination for the presence of dimples, pits, or a sacral fat pad

✓   Scrotal examination to evaluate for epididymitis or epididymo-orchitis

Suggested Work-Up

Urine culture	In infants and young children 2 months to 2 years of age, the urine specimen should be obtained by suprapubic aspiration or transurethral bladder catheterization. The diagnosis of UTI cannot be established by a culture of urine collected in a bag. Older children can provide a clean-catch midstream urine specimen. Criteria for the diagnosis of UTI are presented in Table 46-1.

| Urinary tract ultrasonography | Should be performed on all infants and young children 2 months to 2 years of age with fever and their first documented UTI. May be considered for older children, although the yield is lower |

| VCUG or RNC | VCUG or RNC is recommended for all infants and young children 2 months to 2 years of age with fever and their first documented UTI to detect reflux. May be considered for older children, although the yield is lower |

Additional Work-Up

| Urine dipstick analysis | Urine dipstick analysis can rule out UTI if the result is negative, but a positive result on dipstick testing is insufficient to diagnose UTI |

| Complete blood cell count (CBC), C-reactive protein, and sedimentation rate | Not routinely indicated but may help to determine the presence of a UTI if the clinical picture and urinalysis are equivocal |

| Blood cultures | Indicated for infants younger than 60 days of age |

Method of Collection	Diagnostic Threshold
Suprapubic aspirate	Gram-negative bacilli: any number Gram-positive cocci: more than a few thousand
Transurethral catheterization	10,000 CFU/mL Repeat testing if 1000–10,000 CFU/mL
Clean-catch void in boys	10,000 CFU/mL
Clean-catch void in girls	100,000 CFU/mL Repeat testing if 10,000–100,000 CFU/mL

CFU, colony-forming units.

Table 46-1. Criteria for the Diagnosis of Urinary Tract Infection

References
1. Alper BS, Curry SH. Urinary tract infection in children. *Am Fam Physician* 2005;72: 2483–2488.
2. American Academy of Pediatrics. Practice parameter: the diagnosis, treatment, and evaluation of the initial urinary tract infection in febrile infants and young children. *Pediatrics* 1999;103:843–852.

3. Chang SL, Shortliffe LD. Pediatric urinary tract infections. *Pediatr Clin North Am* 2006;53:379-400.
4. Chon C, Lai F, Shortliffe LM. Pediatric urinary tract infections. *Pediatr Clin North Am* 2001;48:1445.
5. Lin DS, et al. Urinary tract infection in febrile infants younger than eight weeks of age. *Pediatrics* 2000;105:e20.

Index

Printed in the United States
By Bookmasters